W9-CQO-756

ENDORSEMENTS & QUOTES

ENDORSEMENTS & AUTHOR QUOTES

*"It was my privilege to introduce the authors of this book
to each other, Dan Purjes and Scott Stoll, M.D."*
Caldwell Esselstyn, Jr., M.D.

"This book can become responsible for a seismic revolution in health."
Caldwell Esselstyn, Jr., M.D.

*"I hope this book is read and shared far and wide
because it contains the future of healthcare."*
Joel Fuhrman, M.D., author of the bestseller *Eat To Live* and many other books,
President of the Nutritional Research Foundation

*"There is little emphasis on teaching this information in
medical schools and little enthusiasm for it with those
practicing cardiovascular medicine."*
Caldwell Esselstyn, Jr., M.D.

"Dieting simply doesn't work."
Scott Stoll, M.D., co-author

*"It is easy to see that trying to balance 50 million calories
to control weight over a lifetime is nearly impossible."*
Scott Stoll, M.D., co-author

*"For centuries, humanity has searching for the ever-elusive
fountain of youth. It is none other than this whole plant food lifestyle."*
Dan Purjes, co-author

*"Every bite that we put into our mouths has a positive
or negative impact on our cells."*
Scott Stoll, M.D., co-author

"Remember this truth: Your body's natural state is health, not disease."
Scott Stoll, M.D., co-author

"It is never too late to start feeling better."
Dan Purjes, co-author

QUOTES BY STORYTELLERS

"I made the decision to not just lose the weight,
but to gain back my health."
Mary Snyder

"No one ever discussed diet and nutrition with me at all.
Not one doctor ever did that! Nor was it discussed in medical school.
Nor in my residency. How could something so simple as proper
nutrition fix my problems? I couldn't believe it!"
Micha Yu, M.D.

"The thing that gets me is why doctors don't tell patients about things
like this diet before they go in and do surgery."
Jim McNamara

"It was the gift of this book that would become
the lifestyle I always needed."
Colleen Greco Trovato, Editor of Disease Reversal Hope

"If I am the problem, then I get to be the solution."
Adam Sud

"No food feels as good as being pain-free does."
Leila Dehghan, M.D.

"In short, plants saved my life in more ways than one.
Not bad for a former troubled teen, drug addict, alcoholic, ex-hunter,
blue collar worker that decided to give plants a chance."
Will Irving

"The cancer clinic closed my file,
stating that my cancer was undetectable."
Dan Moskaluk

"Healthy blood vessels mean a healthy life!"
Jimmy Conway, M.D.

"A person like me, who is so controlled and rigid, fall hard when
illness hits. I blamed my poor daughter for being the cause
of my illness. I was angry and mad for a long time. But now
I feel healthier than ever before. In some ways, the crazy thing is
that getting sick was the best thing that happened to me.
I realize now that my daughter didn't make me sick. She saved me."
Monica Aggarwal, M.D.

*"I could eat a lot of carbs and not have to worry
about counting calories or restricting my diet."*
Erin Stanczyk

"We started by changing our minds, and the rest followed."
Dan & Sheanne Moskaluk

*"I have learned that it is not illness that defines us
but rather how we respond to it that makes us who we are."*
Monica Aggarwal, M.D.

*"Though no one can go backward and start over, anyone can
start now and make a brand new ending."*
Paul Chatlin

"I believe a rotator cuff tear to be a "heart attack" of the shoulder."
Jimmy Conway, M.D.

*"Change only happens when the pain of not changing
is greater than the pain of changing."*
Emily Boller

*"With my life experience, I should have been dead
or in jail. Now I feel awesome."*
Will Irving

"It seemed like surgery after surgery, and I was ready for it to be over."
Jim McNamara

*"Most physicians don't have either the time or training to sufficiently
educate patients about diet choices."*
Michelle O'Donoghue, M.D.

"One by one, I was able to eliminate all my medications."
Esther Lebeck Loveridge

*"[Surviving terminal cancer], I am not an anomaly.
I eat whole foods, plant-based. That's it."*
Dan Moskaluk

*"We now know that a well-planned vegan diet is healthful for all stages of life,
including pregnancy, breastfeeding, and beyond."*
Erin Stanczyk

"What happened next was beyond remarkable. My doctor assumed there had been a mistake at the lab. He asked to take a blood test again. It was an unheard of dramatic remission, but being healed was just not something we ever considered."
Brooke Goldner, M.D.

"I never knew this could happen. I realized that I could totally do this!"
Jackie Olmstead

"If I was to eat what everyone else was eating, I would suffer what everyone else was suffering."
Colleen Greco Trovato, editor of Disease Reversal Hope

"I knew about being fat, and I knew about losing weight. Both were definitely hard, but only one offered the life I wanted for myself."
Mary Snyder

"I believe that many of us have forgotten what being completely healthy feels like."
Leila Dehghan, M.D.

"It is magical. Now my energy is through the roof. My mind Is clear and vibrant. I no longer need to take allergy pills. I am happy and joyful like never before in my life."
Valeria Popov

"It's really a feeling of independence, because now I feel like I'm fixing myself."
Jim McNamara

"The weight loss continued for a total of three years until I lost not just 70 pounds but 130 pounds."
Esther Lebeck Loveridge

"I had graduated medical school the year before, so it truly never crossed my mind that diet could impact my disease. After all, I would have learned that in medical school, wouldn't I?"
Brooke Goldner, M.D.

"I gained confidence in knowing that being different isn't a bad thing when the common culture in our country is jumping off a cliff regarding heath and wellness."
Marcy Madrid

"For the first time in my life, I'm comfortable with how I look and I don't feel the need to obsess over the numbers on the scale."
Jackie Lopez

DISEASE REVERSAL HOPE!

REAL PEOPLE.
REAL STORIES.

**WRITTEN BY
DAN PURJES
AND SCOTT STOLL, M.D.**

DRH Publishing, LLC
Sarasota, Florida

DISEASE REVERSAL HOPE! Real People. Real Stories.
This edition published in the USA in 2022 by DRH Publishing, LLC

DRH Publishing
5531 Cannes Circle, Suite 703
Sarasota, FL 34231
info@DRHPublishing.com

First edition published on December, 2021.

Authors: Dan Purjes and Scott Stoll, M.D.
Copyright November 15, 2021
The authors have asserted their moral rights.

ISBN #: 979-8-9850982-1-1

No part of this book may be reproduced in any form or by any means without the prior permission in writing from the publisher.

Typeset in December, 2021 by Serff Creative Group, Inc.

First edition printed on December, 2021
Purjes Foundation
PurjesFoundation.org

DEDICATION

*This book is dedicated to each courageous person who wrote
their story and selflessly provided it to be published in this book.
Each and every one of them communicated how, having turned their well-being
and life around, they wanted to help others regain health, vitality,
and happiness through a whole plant food lifestyle.
Their lives are a beacon of hope that lights the path to restored
health and vibrant life.*

Dan Purjes additionally dedicates this book to his wife, Edna ("Ed") Purjes, who brought the light of her life into his life, and to Caldwell Esselstyn Jr., M.D. and his wife, Ann, who brought the wisdom of whole plant foods into his life.

Scott Stoll, M.D., additionally dedicates this book to his wife, Kristen, and to all the pioneering healthcare providers who, moved by compassion for their patients, diligently sought the truth and now lead a global movement of transformation through lifestyle medicine.

"Once you are saved, the only thing left is to help save others."
The Buddha.

DISCLAIMERS

DISEASE REVERSAL HOPE!

Real Stories, Real People.

Medical Disclaimer

This book contains the ideas and opinions of its authors and is solely intended to provide general information. It is not in any way intended to provide specific medical advice, guidance, or act as a substitute for the advice of the reader's own physician or medical professional.

Readers should only seek medical advice from their own physician or healthcare provider, based upon the reader's personal situation, circumstances, conditions, symptoms, diagnoses, or concerns. If the reader desires or requires personal dietary, medical, lifestyle, health, exercise, counseling, or any other assistance, the reader should immediately consult with a competent qualified healthcare professional. At no time should the reader make any adjustments to medication dosages or medical care without the strict guidance of the reader's personal physician.

Before reading this book, please be advised that the publisher and authors specifically disclaim any consequences, direct or indirect, injury, damage, or loss of any kind the reader may incur by following the information, suggestions or guidance provided in this book or by participation in any of the programs listed in this book. The reader should consult with the reader's own physician or healthcare provider before following any of the suggestions or guidance provided in this book, and the reader should follow only the reader's physician's guidance.

Stories Disclaimer

The stories presented here were written by the individuals who submitted their stories to the authors of this book, Dan Purjes and Dr. Scott Stoll. In many, but not all, cases the authors personally know these individuals, having met, or communicated with them directly. The authors edited these stories for grammar and flow but made every effort to leave the stories unchanged as much as possible, to be told in the authentic voice of the storyteller.

The authors of this book, Dan Purjes and Dr. Scott Stoll, made no independent investigation, and therefore provide no representation as to the validity and accuracy of the stories published in this book. The authors personally believe the stories are true and accurate but cannot give any assurance that they are.

All the individuals who contributed their stories for publication in this book signed a non-exclusive copyright release and a final acceptance letter agreeing to the publication of their story. They also granted permission to publish their personal medical and other data as provided by them in their story.

There is no assurance that the disease reversal you read about in these stories will happen to you or in the same way. Converting to a whole plant food diet will undoubtedly improve health, but there is no way to predict in what ways and to what extent. The body is a self-healing organism, but sometimes too much damage has been done in previous years to reverse disease totally. But every step towards health helps.

The authors personally know many people who have reversed chronic diseases to a greater or lesser extent through conversion to a plant-based diet. In some instances, there did not appear to be any improvement in a specific chronic disease, but in all instances, there was improvement in health and general well-being. It is not possible to know what it will do for you until you try it and fully adhere to it for at least 90 days under medial supervision.

TABLE OF CONTENTS

TABLE OF DISEASES

FORWARD
BY CALDWELL B. ESSELSTYN, JR., M.D.

In my journey as a plant-based health practitioner, it was my privilege to introduce the authors of this book to each other: Scott Stoll, M.D., an established leader in the plant-based movement to improve health and avoid disease, and Dan Purjes, a businessman, philanthropist, and visionary committed to enable public and professional awareness of the healing power of plant-based nutrition.

Since finding each other, they have been on an unrestrained pathway of accomplishment. These endeavors include founding the *International Journal of Disease Reversal & Prevention* and merging Plant-based Docs and Plant-Based Doctors, the two leading directories of plant-based nutrition practitioners.

It is my privilege to write the Forward for their latest combined effort: **DISEASE REVERSAL HOPE! Real People. Real Stories.**

These authors have defined an overdue revolution in medicine. Anyone reading this book will recognize in the stories how overwhelmingly powerful and simple it is to protect yourself from chronic disease. Meanwhile pharmaceutical houses and many physicians will nonetheless promote their symptom-treating drugs and interventional therapies, which cannot compete with the curative strength of plants.

While medical entitlements, especially Medicare and Medicaid, are taking this country to the poorhouse, it is chronic illness, the seemingly resistant component to resolution or cure, that is the major culprit.

For example, cardiovascular disease accounts for 45% of Medicare and is expected to cost the country $800 billion per year by 2030, and yet we have known for over 100 years that there are multiple cultures on the planet where cardiovascular disease is virtually nonexistent. They thrive on whole food plant-based (WFPB) nutrition with minimal oils. Dr. Dean Ornish and I have for over thirty years separately proven through experimental studies, which were reported on multiple occasions in the scientific literature, that patients seriously ill with cardiovascular disease may arrest and reverse their illness with WFPB nutrition.

Nevertheless, there is little emphasis in teaching this information in medical schools and little enthusiasm for it with those practicing cardiovascular medicine. Consequently, patients are treated with a plethora of expensive drugs, which have significant side effects, as well as the overuse of stents and coronary by-pass surgery. As none of these therapies address the causation of cardiovascular disease, these patients are left with a lifetime of pain, suffering and recurring illness.

Conversely, for over thirty years, I have enjoyed caring for such patients with WFPB nutrition, avoiding drugs and interventions, making them confident in their own ability to eliminate their disease.

Authors Stoll and Purjes make a similar case that many chronic illnesses will respond to WFPB nutrition approaches to reverse such diseases as diabetes, hypertension, Crohn's disease, ulcerative colitis, rheumatoid arthritis, Lupus, multiple sclerosis, and obesity, to mention a few.

Purjes and Stoll have identified case reports for multiple chronic diseases where the participants themselves tell their story. Each is a saga of disease development, mismanagement with present day remedies, and finally disease resolution as they embraced plant nutrition.

The culmination of all these encounters forms the bastion of enlightened nutritional science that will empower persons to eliminate chronic disease.

This book can become responsible for a seismic revolution in health. It has defined the lifestyle and most specifically the nutritional literacy that can empower the public as the focus of control to annihilate chronic illness.

Caldwell B. Esselstyn, Jr., M.D.
Author of the bestselling book, *Prevent and Reverse Heart Disease*

INTRODUCTION
BY DAN PURJES & SCOTT STOLL, M.D.

"Let food be thy medicine" – Hippocrates

This book contains incredible, inspiring stories by people who reversed terrible, chronic diseases and reclaimed their quality of life, joy, and hope for a better future.

Today, the scourge of chronic diseases is more widespread than any pandemic that has ever afflicted humanity. It is estimated that about two-thirds of all Americans and three billion people globally suffer from at least one chronic disease. Many are dying. Billions of people are suffering unnecessarily and live without hope for a better, healthier future. It is our sincere desire that this book will help many of these people to discover a pathway to a healthier, happier life.

Chronic diseases, as defined by modern medicine, are diseases that progressively get worse over a lifetime, are not curable by medications or medical procedures, are not infectious, and are generally attributable to a combination of lifestyle, aging and genetic factors. Today, chronic diseases are found in every country around the world — diabetes, cardiovascular disease, cancer, hypertension, lupus, rheumatoid arthritis, multiple sclerosis, autoimmune diseases, allergies, digestive ailments, obesity, depression, and many others. And the current medical system doesn't have an answer to this growing tsunami of lifestyle related disease.

AS THE STORIES IN THIS BOOK SHOW, IT DOES NOT HAVE TO BE THIS WAY.

Here are stories by dozens of people, in their own voice, who suffered multiple chronic diseases. In each case they reversed diseases without drugs, surgeries, or medical procedures. They tell you plainly and directly what happened to them — how they suffered from the disease, how they hit the pit of hopelessness, and the steps they took to reverse their disease and climb the ladder of hope and health.

(We define disease reversal as reversing the underlying process that caused the symptoms or the medical findings of a diagnosis, ultimately reaching the established level defined by medical professionals to signify the disease is in remission.)

As amazing as that may seem, there's more. They lost weight until they reached an optimal level, under medical guidance they discontinued medications which had been prescribed for years, regained vitality and energy, and took control of their healthy future. As a bonus, they also greatly reduced their risk of experiencing moderate to severe Covid-19.

There was no magic pill, secret process, unique superfood, or supplement involved. No special procedures or unusual genes involved. They did this by adopting a whole food, plant-based lifestyle, eating as much as they wanted every day, if it was whole plant food. For some people this was very easy, for others it was very hard, but for everyone it was absolutely worth it.

AND IT CAN BENEFIT EVERYONE.

Don't take our word for it. Read the stories yourself. Each story is written by the person in their own authentic voice, and it is true, no matter how incredible. We edited these stories, but we did not write them because we believe it is important to let each person express themselves in their own personal way.

As a result, each story is unique and reads differently than all the others.

The people who wrote the stories in this book are ordinary people. They do not have extraordinary genes or some other unusual physical characteristics that helped them reverse disease. They are just like you. They are just like us.

Interestingly, several of the disease reversal stories in this book were written by physicians about their own chronic diseases. That's right, doctors who themselves suffered from debilitating chronic diseases, including multiple sclerosis, lupus, rheumatoid arthritis, heart disease, diabetes, obesity, and hypertension.

It surprises people to hear that physicians and nurses suffer from the same diseases as their patients. Shouldn't they be healthier, with all their knowledge and access to healthcare?

It surprises people to learn that doctors can get just as sick as everyone else despite years of medical education, training and experience, and access to the latest medical knowledge.

But why should that be surprising? They grew up in the modern era of fast food, stressful work environments, sleepless nights, and invasive technology. They were trained to rely on pharmaceuticals for the treatment of disease. They were not educated about nutrition or the dramatic impact it has on disease.

"Let food be thy medicine," Hippocrates reportedly said. For many centuries, new physicians took the Hippocratic oath to do no harm to patients intentionally and to follow a code of ethics. But the message of Hippocrates to let food be medicine appears to have been forgotten.

Most physicians receive less than 25 hours of nutritional education during their entire seven to twelve years of medical training. It is no surprise, therefore, that physicians don't understand how to prevent, suspend, or reverse chronic diseases in their own lives — diseases that for the most part are caused by an unhealthy diet and lifestyle.

A significant portion of the education in medical school is focused on pharmaceutical drugs and their safe and appropriate use in disease management. Drug companies fund medical schools and university hospitals with huge amounts of money, paying for clinical studies, conferences, and grants. Blockbuster drugs are proprietary, and they generate billions of dollars of revenue for pharmaceutical companies, so it's natural that they would invest huge amounts of money into medical schools and hospitals.

But there is nothing proprietary about a peach. So, there is little money in funding clinical studies on the health benefits of whole plant food nutrition and its ability to reverse and prevent chronic disease. That's why there are much fewer scientific studies of whole plant food nutrition than traditional medical tools like medications.

There is limited financial benefit for hospitals, clinics, and medical practices to promote a plant-based diet to treat the myriad diseases that afflict humanity today. Reimbursement models favor large volumes of procedures. Angioplasty and stent implantation generate tens of thousands of dollars in fees. Coronary artery bypass surgery generates hundreds of thousands of dollars. Urging patients to convert to a whole plant food diet takes more time and yields lower revenue, but it is the heart of true patient care and is the right thing to do.

This is not meant to suggest that the medical profession is diabolical or dishonest. For the most part, doctors, nurses, and hospitals want to do what's best for their patients and are doing what they were trained to do during their education. The problem is the system that has evolved to over-emphasize drugs, devices, and surgical procedures to treat disease, rather than lifestyle and proper nutrition to prevent and reverse it.

Let's look at another health problem to understand this dilemma. For decades many physicians believed that smoking cigarettes was not harmful to health. In fact, some physicians actually participated in advertising that promoted smoking as a healthy way to reduce stress. As a group, doctors had one of the highest percentage smokers of any profession.

Despite the fact that thousands of research studies highlighted the dangers of smoking, including 5 large studies in the 1950's that linked tobacco with lung cancer, despite the Surgeon-General of the United States placing a warning label on cigarette packs in 1965, and despite millions of deaths from adverse consequences of smoking, many doctors continued to smoke. It was only years later, in the 1970s, as sentiment increasingly shifted against smoking, that doctors began to give up smoking themselves and urged their patients to do so as well. And that is when many people stopped smoking.

The industrialized Western diet and lifestyle are the "tobacco" of our generation. There have been thousands of scientific studies repeatedly demonstrating that diets high in processed food and animal products are averse to health, and that whole plant-based foods are beneficial.

Yet doctors are reluctant to recommend a nutrient-dense, whole food plant-based diet to their patients, perhaps because so few of them are plant-based themselves. Most would support the premise that eating more whole plant foods leads to a healthier immune system and lower disease risk, but only a small percentage are actively recommending a lifestyle that includes a whole food plant-based diet as an intervention for chronic disease.

While most physicians support the premise that a healthier immune system is better equipped to deal with Covid-19 and that whole plant foods promote a healthier immune system, very few urge their patients to convert to a whole plant food lifestyle. Why? Could it be because so few of them are plant-based?

(In June 2021, the British Medical Journal, a highly respected peer-reviewed journal, published new research on 3,000 front-line Covid-19 workers showing that those on a plant-based diet had a 73% lower probability of having moderate to severe Covid-19. Kim, Hyunju, et al. "Plant-based diets, pescatarian diets and COVID-19 severity: a population-based case–control study in six countries." BMJ Nutrition, Prevention & Health *(2021): bmjnph-2021.)*

Modern medicine treats the symptoms of chronic disease, not its root cause. Medications and procedures predominantly manage the symptoms and may even slow the progression of disease, but they do not identify or reverse the root cause. Therefore, chronic diseases commonly progress over time and require stronger dosages and additional medications to treat worsening conditions that are caused by unhealthy lifestyle choices. Prescribing a whole plant food diet to reverse chronic disease, rather than medications or procedures, runs counter to the way medicine is practiced today in most places. Sadly, most healthcare providers know very little about nutrition's impact on disease remission and reversal.

If someone walked into a doctor's office with a sharp, stabbing pain in their foot from a nail in their shoe, the physician could either prescribe medication to alleviate the symptom of pain or they could remove the nail from the bottom of the shoe. Modern conventional medicine takes the former approach by prescribing medications for the "pain of the nails of lifestyle diseases." Lifestyle medicine pulls the nail out.

It is time that medicine pivots to treat the root cause of lifestyle diseases. The good news is there is a scientifically validated pathway to improved health, vitality, and disease reversal. It begins with an inspired decision to change what is on our plates every day. The cumulative power and global impact of a plant-based plate, better sleep, less stress and more activity are far beyond what most people would imagine. The stories in this book are a visible representation of what can be possible when that power is harnessed and applied every day.

CHANGE YOUR PLATE, TRANSFORM YOUR LIFE.
How to Use this Book

Each story in this book is accompanied by an introduction to the contributor. Most of the writers have provided photos of themselves as well as contact information. Many of them are active now in the plant-based world, with commercial or with non-profit activities aimed at spreading the word about plant-based health. They tell everyone they meet that a whole food, plant-based diet is the way to live. Feel free to contact them directly. They would love to hear from you.

We created two tables of contents for you, the reader. One lists the chapters and stories in this book. The second is a table of contents of diseases; it lists chapters by diseases and the stories that tell of their reversal. Many stories are about multiple diseases, so you may find the same story listed multiple times.

This book is for you. Everyone who shared their story participated so that someday you can tell your own story of disease reversal. Read this book and learn how to take control of your health.

There is no assurance that the disease reversal you read about in these stories will happen to you or in the same way. Converting to a whole plant food diet will undoubtedly improve health, but there is no way to predict in what ways and to what extent. The body is an excellent self-healing organism, but sometimes too much damage has been done in previous years to reverse it all. But every step towards health helps.

Every journey begins with but one step – take that step and read this book. Find ailments like yours in this book. Read how those diseases were reversed. Transition to a whole plant food lifestyle and open the door to a new world of health and vitality.

We would love to hear your story and possibly publish it in a future volume of **Disease Reversal Hope!** Please send your story to: *info@DiseaseReversalHope.org*

We believe most people know at least one person who is suffering from chronic disease. This book will set them on the path of healing and help them take that first step. Please give them a copy of this book and the gift of health.

If you are interested in ordering a large volume of copies for an organization or health care community, please email *info@DiseaseReversalHope.org* with your inquiry.

If you are looking for a whole food, plant-based physician or healthcare professional please visit **Plantbaseddocs.com**. This is a global directory that helps people who are suffering from chronic disease find a plant-based physician who suits their preferences and can guide them into the healing world of nutrition-based health.

All proceeds from the sale of this book and future related books, and from the sale or rental of the films based on the books, net of expenses, will be contributed to non-profit organizations that promote whole plant foods.

THANK YOU FOR READING THIS BOOK AND TELLING OTHERS ABOUT IT.

FROM PILLS TO PLANTS
ADAM SUD

Conditions: Addiction, depression, anxiety, obesity, diabetes, hypertension, ADHD, erectile dysfunction

Adam Sud was addicted to food and drugs. He weighed 340 pounds and had diabetes. He was so severely depressed that he attempted suicide at the age of 30. Then he decided to take responsibility for his life. He converted to a whole food, plant-based lifestyle. He lost 170 pounds and became a coach for the Mastering Diabetes Program, a non-profit organization that has helped thousands of people reverse diabetes. Also, Adam believes that a whole plant food lifestyle can help reverse depression, anxiety, and other mental challenges. Adam is the founder and Executive Director of the non-profit organization, "Plant-based for Positive Change," which is conducting a scientific study to demonstrate the positive effects of a plant-based diet on addiction and recovery.

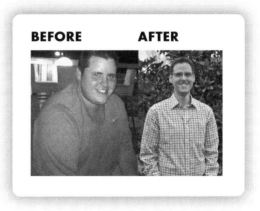

BEFORE   AFTER

@plantbasedaddict & **@plantbasedforpositivechange**

I LIKE TO DESCRIBE MY STORY AS A JOURNEY FROM PILLS TO PLANTS.

My name is Adam Sud, and I am a 7th generation Texan and a Jew. I grew up eating burgers and barbeques, bagels and blintzes, and of course fried chicken on Friday nights. That was a tradition in my family growing up. I like to describe my diet as the Standard American Diet wearing cowboy boots with some chutzpah. I had great friends, played sports and had a great childhood.

However, growing up I struggled with my relationship to food. I can remember being a closet eater as early as age 10. I believed that there must be something wrong with me for wanting "bad" food so badly. I believed I was broken, and because of that I needed to hide this behavior from the world, so no one would know exactly how broken I was.

I was also diagnosed with ADHD at a young age and put on Ritalin. A doctor told me that there was something about me that didn't work properly, but as long as I took this pill, no one would know. From that point on whenever I saw something about myself that others didn't like or that others didn't agree with, I looked for a substance to fix it.

In high school I started to abuse Adderall. I absolutely loved it! Adderall seemed to solve all my problems. It gave me endless energy and I could party all night Friday and Saturday, and then be able to stay up all night Sunday to get my work done. It allowed me to lose the extra weight I had in high school.

During this time, I was struggling with my relationship with my father. I never believed that I was enough of the person he wanted me to be. But when I was on Adderall, I felt like I was finally able to be that person. I believed the more I took this drug, the more it made me the person I wanted to be. I was hooked.

By the time I was in college things had begun to spiral out of control. I needed to take more and more Adderall each time and soon it became more important to me than my classes, my friends, and even my family. I was buying from friends and going through my prescriptions faster and faster each time. Needing the drug had become the most important thing in my life. I ended up dropping out of school and moving back to my hometown of Austin, Texas.

I told my parents it was for a job. But it was really to be back around all my dealers. This is when it all fell apart for me. I lost the job, I avoided my friends, and I was treating my parents like an ATM. I would only see them in order to borrow money or blame and shame them for everything wrong in my life.

I started doctor shopping. This is when you have multiple doctors prescribing the same medication without them knowing about each other. I was forging prescriptions and buying drugs on the street. I had become incredibly depressed and isolated, and I developed a secondary addiction to fast food.

When I say I was a fast-food addict, let me tell you what I would eat in a single day. I would start with 4 - 6 egg-and-cheese breakfast tacos with potatoes. Then for my first lunch, I would get a super-sized, double-quarter pounder meal from McDonald's with an extra double-quarter pounder, since one was not nearly enough. Then for my second lunch, I would go to Whataburger and order the honey-BBQ chicken strip sandwich meal. Then for dinner, I would order an extra-large pizza from Papa-John's with beef on top and a side of the chicken strips. This was still not enough. At around 2:00am I would hit Whataburger again, this time for three of their "breakfast on a bun" sandwiches. I would also drink anywhere from 10 - 20 sodas a day.

My weight reached almost 350 pounds. I was constantly self-conscious about my weight. It didn't help that with my 50-inch waist, the only place I could shop for pants and shorts was at a store called "Casual Male XL." Shopping for clothes would leave me feeling humiliated and disgusted with myself. I would come home from the store, take off my shirt, and look at myself in the mirror in my filthy apartment. I would stare at my body, scanning the entirety of my obese stomach with utter hatred. Seeing every stretch mark, every lump, and every sore that on my body would bring me to tears, anger and self-hatred.

The hatred for my physical appearance would grow and grow until I would begin to punch myself as hard as I could in the stomach, over and over again. Again and again, I would punch myself, while screaming, "I hate you!" with every punch, until I would start to cry. I would stare at the red marks left on my stomach from the beating I had just inflicted upon myself. Collapsing to the floor in defeat, I realized that no matter how hard I hit, I could never win.

I was never comfortable in any social situation without being high, and when I was high it was very noticeable. I was super addicted to Adderall. The average dosage is around 20 mg per day, but I was taking 450 mg in a 24hr period. I was miserable and angry at everyone and everything. I wasn't working because no one would hire an obese, smelly, dirty, college drop-out, drug addict. I was running out of money. I knew that I was heading towards the day when I would be living on the street. That day was very close. I had literally spent every cent I had or could get on drugs and drug-fueled compulsive shopping.

I can still remember the feeling of hopelessness when I would look at myself in the mirror and know that I had a serious problem but was too scared to do anything about it. It was a crippling feeling to know that the drugs and food were destroying my life, but the idea of giving them up, giving up the only things that brought me comfort, was too terrifying to accept.

It was around this time that Whole Foods established a partnership with Rip Esselstyn and his Engine 2 Plantstrong line of plant-based food products. Rip, the son of Dr. Caldwell Esselstyn, Jr., the author of Prevent and Reverse Heart Disease, was a lieutenant in the Austin Fire Department. He launched the Engine 2 line of plant-based foods as a way of getting his Engine 2 firehouse team to convert to a plant-based diet, lose weight, and get healthier. The amazing results attracted the attention of the media. Whole Foods then decided to carry Rip's plant-based products. Whole Foods also offered a week-long Immersion program to help people learn how to adopt a plant-based diet. My Dad, who had been part of Whole Foods since its beginning, saw this as an opportunity to help me and asked that I go. So, I did.

I went to the Immersion, but for no other reason than I knew my father would continue to give me money if I went. While I was there, I was very much a drug addict. To be honest, I was using during the Immersion. But I attended every lecture and learned that by adopting the principles of a plant-based lifestyle, I could prevent and even reverse chronic western disease.

The last night of the Immersion they had a motivational speaker by the name of Dick Beardsley. He talked about how he fought an addiction to painkillers after suffering a series of life-threatening injuries following his career as a world-class marathoner. I listened to this man talk about himself as an addict. The way he treated people and himself, and remembered thinking, "He's talking about me." I wanted so badly to walk up to this man and admit for the first time that I was a drug addict and I needed help, too. Unfortunately,

I wasn't desperate enough to admit to my addiction or to change my diet. I chose the path of fear.

Well, that desperation would come a year later. Sitting on my couch, I had a thought that nothing is ever going to get any better. I was 30 years old, I had already developed erectile dysfunction, and I had given up all hope. I thought I should just spare myself and everyone else the misery I was causing. On August 21, 2012, I attempted suicide by overdose. I ended up lying on the floor, unconscious, surrounded by fast food garbage and empty pill bottles, and in a puddle of my own vomit. Almost dying at the age of 30 from a life of self-hatred, and self-abuse.

Luckily, I regained consciousness and I took a hard look at my life. Suddenly, I had a realization. If I didn't radically change my life, I would wreck the people closest to me. My mom who inspired my imagination and taught me to dream, my dad who taught me the importance of integrity and being selfless and who showed me through his actions what it means to be an honest man, my twin brother who is literally my other half, and with whom I have shared a closeness like with no other person, and my sister who is, well, she is my jewel. I saw these people spending the rest of their lives asking themselves why I needed to eat and drug myself to death.

I also realized that I had received a second chance by surviving. I was going to make sure this would never happen again. I picked up the phone and called my parents. When they answered I said the three words that would change my life forever, "I need help." Two weeks later they were by my side as I checked myself into rehab.

During my first 48 hours in rehab I was searched, drug tested, medically tested, and psychologically tested. I had to do a full body examination with a doctor, which for me, at almost 350lbs, was humiliating. I can recall crying myself to sleep that night. The doctor called me into his office a day later. I walked into his office and sat down across from him. He had a very serious and concerned look on his face. I started to get a knot in my stomach. He looked at me and told me that my fasting blood glucose was over 350 (normal is under 100) and my blood pressure was through the roof. I was diagnosed that day with type 2 diabetes, high cholesterol, and high blood pressure.

In fact, my blood pressure was so high that it had to be monitored every morning before I was allowed to leave the dorms. I was put on multiple prescription medications for type 2 diabetes, high blood pressure, and high cholesterol. Along with antidepressants, mood-stabilizers, ADHD medications, anxiety medications, and sleeping medications. I remember feeling utterly disgusted and ashamed. I finally had to take responsibility for my life and all I wanted to do was quit. I wanted to give up and leave rehab. I thought all I was going to have to do was get off the drugs, which was terrifying enough. But now I was faced with the fact that just getting sober was not enough to save my life.

After talking to my parents on the phone they helped me come to an amazing realization, "If I am the problem, then I get to be the solution." Because of the plant-based immersion, I knew exactly what I needed to do. These were lifestyle diseases that are completely reversible through lifestyle change.

Unfortunately, in rehab you don't have a lot of control of what you eat. You pretty much eat what they serve. I left rehab off the Adderall but on medications for chronic disease and behavior/mood disorders. I entered a sober living house, including drug tests, five hours a day in therapy, and unfortunately, a kitchen stocked with foods that were killing me as quickly as the Adderall had been. I remember thinking to myself, "I might leave here sober but not healthier." I needed to take charge of my life and change my diet.

Now in the beginning of my transition, I made oil-free egg white veggie scrambles to allow me to develop a taste for the veggies. The reason I did this was because along with having to get off the drugs, this was the most discomfort I was able to handle at that time. Then, I transitioned to eating an entirely plant-based diet. This was no easy switch. I cried in the company of people eating pizza and burgers every day. The first few weeks were very difficult, and I was struggling.

Then I read a book by Dr. Doug Lisle and Alan Goldhammer called *The Pleasure Trap: Mastering the Hidden Force That Undermines Health and Happiness.* What I learned from this book was what I have come to believe is the one invariable truth to lifestyle change and recovery. In order to successfully change my life, I had to "be comfortable being uncomfortable."

I knew that if I could just stick with it, I wouldn't always feel deprived, that someday I would not just tolerate but enjoy my changed lifestyle. And I knew that would only happen if I were committed every day to my recovery and learn to make the daily choice between what I want now and what I want most. What I wanted most wasn't to lose weight, reverse my diabetes, and get off the drugs. Of course, I did want to lose weight, reverse my diabetes, and get off drugs, but those weren't my "why." Those things showed me what really mattered most in my life, what I loved enough to be willing to be "comfortable with being uncomfortable."

For me, the "why" was to finally be able to be with my family and not try to take things from them. To be with my family and instead of wanting to use them, simply wanting to just be with them. I told myself that I was not going to try to hate my way out of a destructive life but love myself into a positive one.

Within three to six months, I had completely reversed my Type-2 diabetes, high cholesterol, high blood pressure, and erectile dysfunction. In 10 months, I lost over 100 pounds and within one year I was off every medication prescribed in rehab, including the mood stabilizers, antidepressants, anxiety medication, sleeping medication, and ADHD medication. I have lost over 170 pounds.

I learned that when I prepare a meal on a plate that is about health and healing, it is an act of self-love and self-care. For me, it's an affirmation of sobriety and recovery. People always ask me about what I've lost, and I enjoy telling them about the weight loss and the diseases I have reversed. But my story is not one of loss. What's most profound is what I have gained. Early morning jogs around the lake with my dad, and a real relationship with my parents and the rest of the family. I have found my self-worth and self-confidence, my purpose in life, and the ability to help others. Most importantly my twin brother, Bobby.

Bobby moved into my place in Los Angeles in January 2016 to start his own plant-strong journey. He was overweight and had Type-2 diabetes. Within 6 weeks, his blood glucose was completely normal and as of today he is under 200 pounds for the first time in 10 years. Since then, my entire family has become whole food, plant-based.

I can honestly say that I am the happiest and the healthiest I have ever been in my life. Everything about the way I live my life has changed. The way that I move through the world, the way people interact with me, and the way I interact with other people, have changed. My certainties about the world have completely changed. Today, I feel closer to my authentic self than ever.

That's what recovery is really about – the search for the authentic self.

I feel grateful to have gone through everything that has happened to me – the addiction, the obesity, the diseases. Even the overdose. It has allowed me to become the person I am today. I have learned that I am not now, nor have I ever been, broken.

A plant-based lifestyle didn't save my life. It has given me the ability to create an entirely new one. It's one that I look forward to living every single day. I firmly believe that the simplest change on your fork can be the most profound change of your life. I know it has been for me.

Adam Sud

FROM MULTIPLE SCLEROSIS TO MARATHONS

SARAY STANCIC, M.D.

Conditions: Multiple Sclerosis

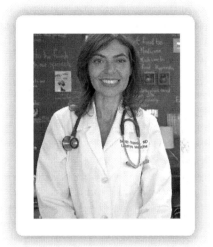

Three years after graduating from medical school, Dr. Saray Stancic was diagnosed with multiple sclerosis. She was told she might be in a wheelchair by her 50s, but instead, that's when she ran the New Jersey Marathon. Her disease and its reversal changed her life and career. In the 1990s, Dr. Stancic had specialized in infectious diseases, hoping to help those with AIDS. Today, she focuses on lifestyle medicine, helping her patients reverse chronic disease. She states, "We must redefine how we practice medicine in the 21st century in order to meet the needs of the changing healthcare landscape."

Get her book, "What's Missing From Medicine: Six Lifestyle Changes to Overcome Chronic Illness" website: **www.drstancic.com** *&* **@drstancic**

In October of 1995, I was, or so I thought, at the top of my game. I was in the third and final year of my Internal Medicine residency and considering a subspecialty. I had been asked by the Chairman of Medicine, a man I deeply admired and respected, to stay on an additional year to complete a Chief Residency. This was an honor, and I accepted it wholeheartedly. In August 1995, I met a wonderful man; he was the one I would someday marry, and we were falling in love. Life was seemingly perfect.

This set the stage for the life-changing events that ensued in the fall of 1995. It was the evening of October 11th, and I was working an overnight shift at the hospital. It was one of those legendary nights, when everything that could go wrong does, and you find yourself in sheer chaos. I was literally sprinting from the emergency room to the intensive care unit and back to the general ward all night. I remember thinking, as I stumbled through that busy night, how incredibly fatigued I felt, much more so than I could recall in the past. Somehow, I kept moving, completing each task with one sole thought in mind, *"Get to your call room and sleep!"* I think it was 3 am when I finally made it to the call room.

As soon as my head hit the pillow, it was lights out in a flash. Predictably, the pager went off shortly thereafter, with requests to address another urgent patient matter. When I lunged forward to answer the call, an extraordinary thing happened. Something had dramatically been altered during that brief nap, and it took my breath away. *I couldn't feel my legs.*

I remember looking down at my lower extremities and acknowledging they were still there. Instinctively, I reached out to touch them, and immediately withdrew as it felt like I was touching someone else. Was I dreaming? I attempted to step down onto the floor to get help, but again immediately retracted when my feet touched the floor. It was as if I was stepping down on a bed of hot coals. I could feel my heart racing, pounding, and fear consumed me. OK, this is real. So, now what? Should I panic, scream, cry, or laugh? Which did I pick? I must confess I don't remember which I chose. Somehow, I got from that bed to the ER. But now, I was the patient.

An emergent MRI was ordered, and they rushed me into the radiology suite. I was told not to move as the length of my body rolled into this machine, leaving me encapsulated, claustrophobic, and increasingly more fearful. The test took two hours to complete, and during that time I began to experience sharp, lancing pain in both legs. The relief of learning the study was complete was immense, but only for a moment. As they moved me out of the MRI suite, I heard the attending radiology physician call out to one of the residents:

"Go get the students. This is a classic case of MS."

What a horrible way to learn of my diagnosis! My heart sank. My eyes welled up. There I was, lying on a gurney, wearing a flimsy hospital gown, vulnerable and fragile, and I just learned I had multiple sclerosis a week after my 28th birthday.

I was admitted to the hospital and started on IV steroids to treat the acute flare-up. I was discharged five days later and told to return in a week to discuss the initiation of modifying therapy for my disease. My doctor explained that this was the key to slowing the progression of this chronic neurologic disabling disorder, and without it I would likely be in a wheelchair within 10 to 20 years. These are very difficult words to hear when you are only 28 years old.

Of course, I would do whatever my doctor asked of me to prevent that from happening. He explained the treatment was very effective but warned it would not be easy. I would have to inject this drug daily. When I asked for how long, he replied "for the rest of your life."

My doctor added that the side effect profile of the drug could be challenging. The side effects included fever, chills, muscle aches, pain, nausea, vomiting, diarrhea, insomnia, hair loss, anorexia, injection site reactions, depression, and suicidal thoughts. Despite all of this, he urged me not to worry as he believed most side effects could be avoided by pre-medicating with ibuprofen before the injection and administering the drug at bedtime. In this way, he predicted, I would sleep through all the side effects. He urged me to start immediately because any delay could worsen my prognosis.

What followed seemed worse than the diagnosis. I would inject the drug at 10 pm and awaken at 2 am with violent shaking, chills, fever, nausea, and more. After a few weeks, I didn't think I could do this much longer. I phoned my doctor to let him know I was calling it quits. Right away, he explained this wasn't an option and reminded me of the wheelchair in case I had forgotten. He said he understood what I was going through and offered a remedy. He explained that the side effects of this drug could be treated with other drugs. So, when I couldn't sleep, I was given a prescription for Ambien; when I couldn't wake up in the morning, I was given a prescription for Provigil, an amphetamine-like drug; and when I became depressed because my life was unravelling, I was given a prescription for Prozac. By the time I was in my early 30's, I had become dependent on nearly a dozen drugs to get through a routine day. Despite all these medications, my disease progressed, and my quality of life suffered immensely.

Eight years into my diagnosis, I had become dependent on a set of crutches or a cane to get around. I began to lose hope. Then, in 2003, amid what seemed my darkest period, came what I call my *"Aha!"* moment, and it came in the oddest of ways. My secretary walked into my office to deliver the daily mail. On this particular day, she dropped a large stack on my desk. It caught my attention, and when I glanced over at the top of the stack, I saw a journal, and on its cover, I saw the words *multiple sclerosis* and, of all things...*blueberries.*

What in the world could blueberries have to do with MS?

Intrigued, I dropped all else, and turned to the article. Frankly, it was disappointing. A poorly constructed study, where they fed half the MS patients a diet enriched with blueberries while the other half consumed their regular diet. The study concluded that there were benefits to the patients who ate the berries and suggested the anti-inflammatory qualities of the blueberry may very well have something to do with the benefits seen.

What???!!!

I remember sharing the study with a colleague on that day. He laughed, and so did I; but there was something about this silly little blueberry study that I could not get out of my head. It wasn't that I thought eating blueberries was going to miraculously improve my MS. A much more important question surfaced from that line of thinking:

Could there be a connection between diet and disease?

Well, if anyone could answer that question, you'd think I'd be able to. After all, I was a physician.

Four years of medical school, four years of residency, and another two years as a subspecialist — that was a decade of higher education in the field of medicine, and I couldn't think of any examples in which my professors, mentors or educators had ever connected the two dots of diet and disease. If this had been important, it would have been covered in medical school. But it wasn't.

Nevertheless, I remained curious. Maybe it was because I was desperate. I decided to explore this question carefully and methodically. I turned to the scientific literature looking for answers, via PUBMED, the medical search engine. I entered terms like *multiple sclerosis* and *diet, chronic disease,* and *diet*...and what I got back was nothing short of remarkable.

One of the first articles I came across was written by Dr. Roy Swank and published in the *New England Journal of Medicine* in 1952. Dr. Swank, a physician who was the first head of neurology at Oregon Health Sciences University, was an early researcher in the link between MS and diet. In one of his research publications, Swank wrote about the incidence of MS in Norway, a country with one of the greatest burdens of MS worldwide.

Interestingly, Swank noted that the highest rates of MS in Norway were occurring in the inland farming community where large amounts of animal foods containing saturated fat were consumed, as compared to coastal areas of the country where people ate large amounts of fish, rather than meat. Based on this recognition, he hypothesized saturated fat was playing a role in the pathogenesis of multiple sclerosis.

Swank did not leave this solely to hypothesis; he went on to treat patients diagnosed with MS with a low fat, plant-based diet. In fact, he followed 140 plus patients over decades, and ultimately concluded in an article published in 1990 that those who adhered to his diet had significantly less disability and mortality. Of those who survived, 95% remained physically active.

These findings fascinated me and offered a glimmer of hope in what otherwise seemed a desperate situation. Reading Swank's work sparked an intense interest to further understand the impact of diet on MS. I continued to search and digest the peer-reviewed medical literature, which was rich in ample corroborative evidence. As my understanding flourished, I came to realize that diet and lifestyle choices were indeed important and might well be a salvation.

Empowered by this new-found knowledge, I scheduled an appointment to see my doctor. I was eager to share what I had learned. I questioned in my own mind why he had never discussed diet and its potential role in MS outcomes. I presented him with copies of the many articles I had discovered and relayed their content enthusiastically hoping that he would be excited by the potential.

But my enthusiasm and proposal seemed to have the opposite effect than what I had hoped. He immediately sought to dissuade my assertions. He remarked that the only proven and effective approach to managing MS was the treatment he had already offered and implored me to continue the medication as prescribed. He advised me to eat the foods I enjoyed. He added, if I wanted to blame anything for having MS, I could lay blame on my genes because that was why I had MS, and there was nothing I could do about that.

I left this visit feeling quite deflated. Whatever hope I had conjured had been swiftly washed away, but not for long. I replayed his parting words in my mind, over and over again: "It's your genes."

This got me thinking about genetics and wondering if anyone had ever looked at monozygotic twins (identical twins) and multiple sclerosis. Monozygotic twins are very interesting in that there are two separate individuals that have the same exact genetic blueprint. I wondered if twin A had MS, what would be the likelihood that twin B would have MS? You would think it would be close to 100% if the primary cause of MS was genetic in origin. Again, I turned to the scientific literature looking for the answer to this question and found the concordance rates between monozygotic twins was nowhere near 100%. It wasn't even 50%. It was more like 14-33%. This discovery was welcoming and brought with it a rekindled sense of hope. It wasn't just my genes, there were other variables playing a significant role.

It was then that I came to learn of the science of epigenetics, which shows that gene expression is dependent on outside variables. Just because you have a gene for a certain condition doesn't necessarily mean it will be expressed. Genes can be *turned on or off*. Epigenetics describes the variables that are important in modifying gene expression. These are diet and nutrition, physical activity and exercise, alcohol and drugs, smoking, etc. In a nutshell, it's our lifestyle choices that turn genes on or off.

Emboldened by this understanding, I grew confident there was more I could do than just fill a prescription. I realized I needed to implement changes in my own life. I accepted I would not receive the support I so desperately sought from my own doctor, but convinced by the evidence, I made the unconventional and difficult personal decision to responsibly taper off all the medications and, moving forward, I would optimize every aspect of my lifestyle.

The first step I took was changing my diet from the standard American diet, rich in animal sources and processed foods, to a whole food, plant-based diet rich in fruits, vegetables, whole grains, legumes, nuts, and seeds. I began to exercise for the first time in years. At first, I was only able to pedal on a stationary bike for a few minutes before I would experience pain and disabling fatigue. But I persisted, and over time I built strength, stamina, and endurance. I created boundaries around my work life, declining to take on additional projects proposed by others. For the first time in my life, I was putting myself first, above all else.

And do you know what happened? Plain and simple, I started to feel better. It didn't happen in a week or in a month, but over time I began to note a marked improvement in my quality of life. Maybe at first it was something as subtle as I could stay up past the evening news, or on a particular day I would feel comfortable enough to leave my cane in the car.

About two years into my lifestyle change came a memorable day. I had been invited to attend a wedding with my husband. On this day, I did two things I hadn't done in years. I wore heels and danced with my husband. Seemingly trivial to others, but for me it was a huge triumph.

Later that year, my brother came to visit me. This was always a treat, as we live on opposite coasts. He hadn't seen me in some time and was thrilled to note I seemed happier, leaner, and free of my cane. During the visit, we celebrated his recent completion of the LA Marathon, and he shared the exhilaration of crossing the finish line after all the work and training. We toasted my newfound wellness, and toward the end of the conversation, he had the audacity to propose I consider *running a marathon.* I immediately was angered by the suggestion and shot back at him, "I can't run a marathon, I have MS!"

What a wonderful gift he had just given me. My immediate response, to grow angry at him for even suggesting it, dissolved into a peaceful awakening. Until that moment, I had defined myself as this woman living with MS. With that label came so many limitations, things I could do and things I could not do. It was then I realized that this had to end. I would not allow this disease to define me any longer.

The seed had been planted. Over time, I grew more and more confident. I found myself attempting to jog short distances. It didn't go well at first. I would lose balance, fall, scrape my knees, but in time I built up enough courage to try again. There is a nature preserve near my home. There is a small body of water and a path that runs along its edge. If you make it the entire way around, it's a bit more than a mile. It isn't much, but I recall the first time I made it the entire way around without falling or stopping, and I felt invincible. It was on that day I made the commitment to someday run a marathon, a challenge that once seemed so unlikely and beyond reach.

On May 2, 2010, with my family and friends surrounding me, I crossed the finish line at the NJ Marathon. It was an extraordinary moment in my life. Not because I ran a marathon, but because this accomplishment symbolized the fruit that had been borne of my efforts. Somehow, those lifestyle changes which had been dismissed as irrelevant by my physician, had actually been the key to my recovery.

Today, more than 25 years since my MS diagnosis, I am free from medication and disability. I am empowered, as a physician and as someone who has regained control from a disabling disease, to share this healing message with whomever is willing to hear it. I hope there is an audience open and eager to listen. If so, it will all be worth it.

Saray Stancic, M.D.

FROM LIVER TRANSPLANT TO MARATHONS

KELLY THRUSH

Conditions: Alcoholism, food addiction, liver disease, diverticulitis, arrhythmia, obesity

Kelly Thrush was on the brink of death from addictions to alcohol and food. His liver was destroyed, and doctors were concerned that he would destroy a transplant with continued drinking. Two doctors put their reputation on the line for him. He received a liver transplant and stopped drinking. And he converted to a whole plant food lifestyle because that was the best way to take care of the transplant and be healthy. Today, Kelly runs marathons, mentors at several organizations, including alcohol recovery, transplant recovery, and outdoor programs for teens. He says, "I am working on becoming the person I was always meant to be."

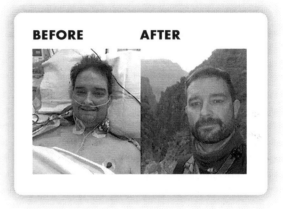

@ThrushKelly

HOW ON EARTH DID I GET HERE?

This is the thought that kept repeating in my mind over and over again; like a broken record, as I sat alone in the hospital room. I was confused. Embarrassed. Ashamed. My dysfunctional relationship with alcohol had destroyed almost everything important to me. It destroyed my marriage. It ruined my relationship with my kids. It destroyed my liver. I was on rocky terms with my family. I had bounced from job to job over the past few years as my addiction had gotten worse. And now, it was literally killing me.

Staring at the ceiling, lost in thought, I was struggling to come to terms with the phrase "end-stage liver failure." I was not supposed to end up in the hospital dying at age 38.

As a teenager I dreamed of being a professional baseball player, or President of the United States. At the very least I was supposed to be a high school teacher and coach the baseball team. I was supposed to be someone people looked up to. I prided myself on my leadership skills, my charm, and my wit. As life would have it, I ended up running bars and restaurants for more than a decade, drinking, and partying most days well into the wee hours of the morning, only to come home, take a nap, wake up and do it all again.

Instead of all my aspirations as a teenager, I was lying in a cold, stale hospital bed, hoping no one would tell my friends and family where I was.

"I can't let them see me like this!" I thought.

Three months earlier, I had been in denial of just how sick I really was. It was a Sunday afternoon, January 7, 2018, when my health began to crumble. We were moving furniture for a buddy of mine. I didn't feel well. I passed it off as being hung over. Or maybe I just hadn't had enough to drink that day. I mean, it was noon and I had only had two drinks. Or possibly it was left over from the flu a couple of weeks prior. I had been sick for the entire month of December. Looking back, I think the reason I was so sick was that my body was beginning to fail me at that point.

There were signs of my disease as early as the summer before. Jamie, my lady, and I were coming back from visiting her family in California. That morning I got sick. We had just finished breakfast when I couldn't keep it down any longer. It couldn't have been more than a few yards outside of the restaurant door when I scurried to find the closest bush and let it all out. Coming up from the bushes, wiping my mouth, I joked and laughed, "where did that come from?"

I chuckled, embarrassed about what had happened. I knew damn well what it was from, but I wasn't going to say it. If I did utter the words out loud, it would mean I should probably not drink that day. No way I was going to let that happen. So, I shrugged it off and convinced myself it would pass and be better by the time we arrived back in Arizona. As the next couple of hours passed, I had to pull the car over. I couldn't drive any longer. Jamie was going to have to finish the trek home. The pain in my abdomen was undeniable. It was this gut-wrenching cramp, just above my belly button and below my sternum that keeled me over. As time passed, it was getting worse. I couldn't sit in the front seat any longer. I had to lay down.

"Jamie, pull over" I whispered. "I have to go to the back seat."

As I crawled behind the passenger seat, she pleaded that I go to the hospital. I convinced her it was nothing. Jamie had no idea that years before I had bouts with diverticulitis. In 2012, my diverticulitis got so bad that it landed me in the hospital a few times. The result was a partial colectomy--I ended up having one third of my colon removed.

Diverticulitis is caused by poor diet. I was most definitely the king of poor diets. Greasy, fatty, and highly processed foods were on the menu every day of my adult life. Those foods can create inflammation in the wall of the large intestine. The inflammation can lead to infections in pouches of the intestines and to abscesses. In my case those abscesses ruptured and needed to be surgically removed.

Sitting in the back of the car writhing in pain, I knew the real reason I did not want to go to the hospital. Why? Because if I sat in front of a doctor, he or she would tell me I drank too much. I wasn't going to let that happen. So, I toughed it out for the next few hours. By morning the cramping had subsided, and I was back to my regular schedule.

Six months later, on Monday, January 8, 2018, I felt a bit worse but manageable. Tuesday the 9th I was at work when one of my employees asked me, slightly tongue in cheek, "Kelly, are you dying?" Slightly embarrassed and taken aback, I smirked and sarcastically responded, "Am I die … dying? No, I am not dying. Get back to work." It wasn't until the next day, Wednesday, January 10, 2018, that everything came to a head. In the middle of the afternoon, I didn't feel well. But I ignored it. I was truly in denial. My boss met me as I came out of my office and told me in no uncertain terms that I was going to the hospital. My response?

"I can't go to the hospital," I said. "I have too much to do today." I have this, that and the other to do. I listed them all out on my fingers. She paused and looked at me and gave me three choices. She mimicked me and listed the options on her fingers: "Kelly, you can find a ride, I can give you a ride, or I can call the ambulance."

I thought to myself, "I look that bad?"

Unbeknownst to me, I had become jaundiced. My skin was yellow. My eyes were yellow. I refused to see any of it. The chef, who is a good friend of mine, came out of the office and held up a yellow post-it notes next to my face for comparison. "You look like this color," he said in jest. None of us knew how sick I was, just that I was sick and needed to go, and go now.

As stubborn as I was, and truly doing my best not to sit in front of a doctor, I still didn't go to the hospital. Instead, I drove myself 40 minutes toward home to go to the small urgent care clinic next to our house. I walked in and the doctor looked at me and said "Why are you here? I can't help you. You need to go to a hospital. Now."

I did. The next few weeks I went to a few different hospitals. I continued to get worse. My liver was shutting down. At this point my kidneys were also shutting down and my abdomen was filling with fluid. Each day I was becoming a deeper shade of yellow. My ammonia levels were reaching points that I would have delusions and hallucinations. I couldn't pee and it hurt when I did. My urine would come out the same color as cola and it felt as thick as cola too. The doctors tried a few things, different procedures to see if they would help me.

One being paracentesis. This is when the doctors would stick a large needle in my abdomen to drain the fluid that had built up. They would take the greenish-yellow Mountain Dew looking fluid out of me by the liters. Multiple liters at a time. This would work for a few days until I would fill up again and must have it drained again. We did this rinse and repeat type procedure, I don't know how many times. We saw multiple doctors and specialists. Many of them told us there was nothing they could do for me. I was too sick. I was too far gone. I needed to get my affairs in order.

Jamie would not take this as an answer. I will say this phrase many more times in life; "Thank God for Jamie." Sitting in the office of one of the liver specialists we visited, he looked at us and said he could not help us. Jamie politely stood up from her chair, responded with "that's not good enough" and pushed my wheelchair out of the room. I truly would not be here if it was not for her.

I finally ended up in a university hospital in mid-February. It was here I met the team that would eventually save my life. But even in this hospital the doctors were not sure they could help me. Here was the dilemma. A full liver transplant seemed to be the only option for me. But the issue for that solution was twofold:

1. Even if I got put on the transplant list, and even if they were able to find me a viable liver, was I too sick for a transplant? There are multiple factors that go into a transplant. One of them is that you must be the right amount of sick. If you are too sick you won't survive the surgery and your body would not be strong enough to endure the trauma. If you are not sick enough, you will be put lower on the list as people with more immediate concern would be addressed first. It is a delicate balancing act.

2. Most importantly, organs are hard to come by. So even if they found a liver, even if I survived the surgery, why would the team give a perfectly good organ to an alcoholic? The fear being that within a short period of time I would simply fall right back into my old habits and waste away my life and liver ... again.

I didn't blame them. They were right. There were plenty of deserving candidates out there and nothing in my life's history gave them any indication I would appreciate what the transplant team was trying to do for me. I had been drinking every day for the past 18 years or so. The only reason I had stopped the past two months was because I had landed myself in the hospital.

Over the years there were so many reasons and moments I should have stopped. The countless fights I had with my former wife about my drinking. The fact is, it destroyed my marriage. My kids who witnessed me drunk, passed out or stumbling on holidays. Not being able to read them bedtime stories because I couldn't concentrate on the pages. My DUI. Spending time in jail as a result. That would have been a great time to stop. Hell, I was nine days sober when I got out. The year I spent sober in 2016. That was good momentum. Why didn't I keep it going? The embarrassment and pain I caused my loved ones over the years. The list goes on and on.

Why should the transplant team have any faith that this time was any different?

Yet, there were two doctors who specifically put their reputations on the line for me. They went to bat for me. They put a plan together and convinced the transplant team I was worth the risk. To this day I am not sure what they saw in me. Why did they decide that this time was different? In order to be put on the transplant list there are many requirements the patient has to complete in order to be eligible. In my case, I had to be sober for a year and attend SMART Recovery meetings. (SMART Recovery is like Alcoholics Anonymous. Same destination, different vehicle). The fact is I was too sick and could not wait a year. At this point I didn't have a month, let alone a year.

Finally, I was put on the list and moved to the top. The day the team found a liver for me could not have come at a better time. I was told the good news in the afternoon. I was prepped for surgery and wheeled down to the ICU. It was right then that my body began to crash. In retrospect I have a theory as to why I crashed so quickly that day. I believe, deep down, on a subconscious level my body was holding on as tight as it could for the news the doctors had found a liver. Once that happened, my body simply exhaled and figuratively said "we can't hold on any longer." While in the ICU, I began bleeding. From anywhere and everywhere it was possible to bleed.

From my insides I was coughing up blood. I was puking blood. I had uncontrollable bleeding out of my nose. Thank God for Jamie. She has been with me the entire time. She is a saint in every sense of the word. She sat with me bedside in the ICU holding a bucket that I would bleed into every few minutes, dumping out the bucket with tears streaming down her face as I bounced in and out of consciousness. To put it into perspective, I had over 20 blood transfusions before I went into surgery. The ICU nurse told Jamie, "If this doesn't happen in the next few hours, he is not going to make it."

I was no longer simply dying. I was actively dying.

In the first 10 seconds after the surgery, I opened my eyes to a wave of emotions that came over me that are impossible to describe. I never know what words to use to truly do them justice. Still hooked up to the ventilator and to countless tubes and machines, I was filled with pure and utter gratitude. I had made it to the other side. I was still alive. I had gratitude for the doctors and team that had spent the last few months working on me, for having faith in me. Thankful for my family who, through all of this, was standing by my bedside. All of whom were huddled around me with tears and smiles as I came to.

And as wonderful as the gratitude that filled me was, the guilt that accompanied it was overwhelming. My poor choices in life damn near killed me. It put my family through pain I will never truly understand. I had caused much wreckage and suffering over the years. How was it possible that I am still here?

"I don't deserve it" I thought.

I could not have one thought without the other. They were an interwoven tapestry of emotions that were unshakable. Why was I able to live that day? My donor didn't. There is a mother out there somewhere who lost her baby that day. But my mom stands here holding my hand misty-eyed and smiling down at me. How is that fair? That is a question I still grapple with to this day.

The road to recovery for me was a difficult one. I had multiple procedures after my transplant. Internal stitches popped out and I began to bleed internally. I was immediately rushed back into the operating room to repair the damage. After I was discharged, infection set in and landed me back in the hospital for another surgery, and a few more weeks of hospital stay.

Once I arrived home the final time, I was very weak. I was nothing but skin and bones. One of the complications of my disease is that when the liver ceases to work properly, the body consumes any protein it can find. In my case, it consumed my muscle mass. I couldn't walk on my own. I needed a walker for short distances and a wheelchair for longer ones. I couldn't shower on my own. If I fell, I could not get back up. Someone would have to come and get me off the floor. I had 24-hour care following my transplant surgery.

When I left the hospital the transplant team gave me a huge binder with all the dos and don'ts for the months to come. It listed keeping track of my health including the exercise routine I should keep and the diet I should maintain. I was to eat a very well-rounded diet. It recommended a low sodium – high protein diet as I healed. I needed to watch my sugars, fats, and water intake. I was diligent about it for months.

As the weeks went on, I was on a mission to recover, and quickly. Being a bit stubborn is both a blessing and a curse. On the one hand, my stubbornness was to blame for how I got myself into this mess in the first place. On the other hand, it was helping me recover and become a better, more well-rounded human being in the process.

I began with small goals. First, I was going to get the mail from the mailbox. Each day I would walk, with my walker and in my house shoes, to the mailbox and back. Next step was to the neighbor's house. Then to the next neighbor's house. So it went, until after only a few weeks I could walk around the block.

Just a few short weeks after my surgery we took our youngest son out for his 8th grade pictures. We were in a national park in the foothills just below the mountains near our house. It is a picture-perfect backdrop for school pictures. When walking down toward the main gate we took the handicap accessible ramp. It was a longer, winding path down towards the entrance to the park. I did not bring my walker that day and was getting stronger on my outings. After about an hour we finished up the photos.

Good! I was beginning to get a bit tired. As we headed toward the ramp back to the parking lot I glanced to my right. It was only 17 stairs back to the car. I looked to the left at the ramp then back to the right and the stairs. And then to Jamie. She let down her shoulders and shook her head no.

"Let's take the ramp," she said. Jamie already knew what I was thinking. I said, "Nope, I am taking the stairs. It's only 17 steps and it is a long way back up that ramp."

"Please," Jamie pleaded.

I shook my head no. We went back and forth a few times, and I finally said, "I am taking the stairs, AND I am not going to use the handrail."

Jamie conceded. She knew I had my mind made up. When I reached the top, it was as if I had won the gold medal at the Olympics. I yelled at the top of my lungs "Woooooo!!!" and pumped my fists in triumph.

At this point I found myself being drawn to the mountains. I would go for hikes. Partly for the physical health benefits, but mostly for the mental health benefits. I liked the solitude. I enjoyed being in nature. I would often pick the trails less traveled. It would be only myself and my dog. We might not see another human being for the entire day. I did not know it at the time, but the hikes were becoming part of what would eventually turn into mindfulness practice. They began to get longer and more challenging. Higher up the mountain I would go, and further into the bush.

Finally, one morning in October of 2018, I was hiking to the top of one of the ridge lines. It was spectacular. I wanted to share it with my sister. I called her to show her the view. She was amazed at where I was and said, "You should run a half marathon with me next month."

My first response was, "What? Are you nuts? There is no way I can run 13 miles." She then asked me quietly, "How long was the hike today?"

"14 miles," I answered.

The next day I signed up to run my first half marathon. Until that point in my life, I had never registered for any race. Not a 5k, let alone a half-marathon.

I decided that in the following months I would ride the Tour de Tucson. This is a well-known bicycle race around the city. I decided I was going to ride the 100-mile race. Jamie asked, "Shouldn't you start with the 25- or 50-mile race?"

"Probably. But I need to go buy a bike first," I answered. I had already made up my mind. At this point I had a lot of crazy adventure ideas. I dragged my family to go swimming with sharks. We went hiking to unknown places.

I had BIG plans down the road. So, whenever I would say, "Jamie, I've been thinking," she would simply shrug her shoulders, and quietly ask, "What now?"

In early 2020 I began to dive down the rabbit hole of endurance sports. I had ridden the tour for 100 miles, and I had run a couple of half marathons, but I wanted to do more. My health seemed to be pretty good, though I had slipped back into a typical American diet over the past couple of years.

I started reading everything I could about long distance running, craving any information about where the next adventure would take me. I noticed a lot of those athletes had something in common besides running. They were vegan.

I consumed everything I could about a whole food, plant-based diet. I watched documentaries, listened to podcasts, and read multiple memoirs about people who had a very similar story to mine. Finally, one day I came home and said "Jamie, I have been thinking." Her shoulders slumped and she simply looked at me. "I am going vegan," I said. Confused, she looked at me and asked "When?"

I replied "Tomorrow."

She was nervous. Not once in the big liver binder of the do's and don'ts, did it say that a WFPB diet was the way to go. In fact, it talks extensively about the different types of meats you should and shouldn't eat as a transplant patient. Remember, I had a poor diet pretty much my entire life. I had been a carnivore my whole life. So, Jamie and I compromised. I would wait to go 100% vegan until I spoke with the dietician on the transplant team. I made the appointment the very next day.

In the couple of weeks that followed, I was for the most part, vegan as I waited for my appointment. When the day finally came, I met with the dietician. I explained my past, I explained my goals, I explained why I wanted to go on a whole plant food diet and how I believed it would benefit me. She was all for it!

We talked about numbers and about tracking food. We talked about the seemingly hundreds of ways to get your protein. Good quality protein at that! We talked about the biology of the human body and how animal flesh interacts with it and the reaction it causes. She was gung ho. I was gung ho. I have been gung-ho and all in ever since!

Going plant based has been one of the best decisions I have ever made. It was a matter of just two weeks before I started to feel the benefits. I slept better. I woke up better. My thoughts were clearer. My performance at work improved. I lost weight. (I have always struggled with my weight). And in the years since my surgery, I had gained all my weight back with a little extra.

In 2020, during the pandemic, several people put on a few pounds. Not me. I lost 45. Between my new exercise routine and my new relationship with food the pounds simply fell off. Now, I won't lie. There are still the last, stubborn 25 lbs. that need to go. But weight is not my goal. It's a by-product of my journey.

I use food as fuel now. It is not a reward, at least not for the most part. I want to make sure I put in my body what it needs. Since really dialing into my nutrition, I can listen to my body when it speaks to me. I can tell when I have not had enough carbs for the day, or I did not get my protein quick enough after a workout. I can tell when I need to up my sodium intake or I did not drink enough water the day before. I find it truly amazing how the human body responds to the types of fuel you put in it. I mentioned earlier I have big goals on the horizon. In order to accomplish them it is going to take discipline in every aspect of my life. Why not fuel my body with the best of fuels - plants?

To date I have run multiple 5 and 10ks, half marathons and even a full marathon, simply because I wanted to see if I could. I have been rim to rim at the Grand Canyon raising money for a local teen center. We will be heading back there again this year. I will be riding in the Tour de Tucson again in November and another marathon in December. To cap the year off, I am currently training for my first Ultramarathon – a 52.5-mile trek through the mountains southwest of Phoenix.

Keeping my body primed with good nutrition is key. Down the road I will be running 100-mile races, and at some point, I will be hiking the Arizona Trail in its entirety: 800+ miles from Mexico to Utah.

The best part about finding my whole food plant-based diet is it fits seamlessly into my core values. Sitting in the ICU with my family surrounding me, filled with emotions that still make me tear up as I type this story, I made a promise. I have a debt I will never be able to repay. There is no good reason I am sitting here today. My promise? I will earn this gift I have been given, every day, for the rest of my life.

Every day I will treat my body with respect. I will take it on adventures. I will take the person whose liver is sitting inside of me on all those adventures too.

Every day I will help others with their journey. I will hold the hands of people who are waiting for their transplants. I will be there to answer their questions. To guide them through the scariest moments of their lives. To hug them when they need it.

Every day I will mentor others with their own addictions. I have become a facilitator for the SMART recovery program. This program is just one of many I owe my life to.

Every day I will be the man Jamie can love for the rest of her life. I owe her at least this much.

Every day I will be the dad I should have always been for my kids. The dad they can be proud of.

People have mentioned to me how much I have changed over the past three years. My answer to them is simple:

I haven't changed. This is the person I have always been.
I had not allowed myself to be him.

Kelly Thrush

HOW MY DAUGHTER SAVED ME
MONICA AGGARWAL, M.D.

Conditions: Rheumatoid Arthritis

Dr. Monica Aggarwal is an Associate Professor of Medicine in the cardiovascular division of the University of Florida. She developed an advanced form of rheumatoid arthritis after the birth of her third child. Suffering through the horrible adverse side effects of the drugs she was prescribed, Dr. Aggarwal learned first-hand the power of lifestyle medicine and the power of a whole food, plant-based diet to reverse disease.

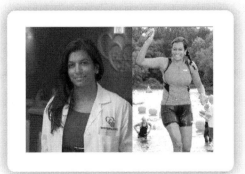

Today, she is the Director of Integrative Cardiology & Prevention at the University of Florida, promoting food as the foundation of healing. Dr. Aggarwal gives presentations throughout the country and has been featured in plant-based magazines. She has published research in major medical journals such as the Journal of the American College of Cardiology and the American Journal of Medicine. Dr. Aggarwal is the author of the book, Body on Fire: How Inflammation Triggers Chronic Illness and the Tools We Have to Fight It.

Website: www.Drmonicaaggarwal.com | **Twitter:** @drmaggarwal
Facebook: drmonicaaggarwal | **Instagram:** drmonicaaggarwal

When I was little, I used to think that I didn't bleed. I was never injured and rarely even received a cut. When my son was born, I remember laughing at myself because of my surprise that when he fell, he would bleed. For some crazy reason, I think we all believe when we are little that we are invincible.

I carried that feeling of invincibility into my 30s. I was a powerhouse. I worked hard and long hours, then came home and crashed, only to wake up and do it again the next day.

I felt I had it all. It is a tricky thing being a career woman, though. We spend our lives studying to reach the top of our game, but then that goal often coincides with the years when we want to have children. I had three children in five years. I poured the same intensity into my children. I nursed them all. I made fresh meals daily, baked their birthday cupcakes and knit their Halloween costumes. I was exhausted. It was a hard life, but I felt that it was a burden I had to accept in order to have it all.

After my third child was born, life changed for me. I recall the time so vividly. I went back to work eight weeks after the baby came. I remember the utter exhaustion of sleeping for three hours, going to work, then running home to nurse, cook meals and start the routine all over again. Every night, my husband would drag me out of one of our children's bedrooms, so I could fall asleep in my own bed, until the next cry woke me up. I was haggard. I felt I had to sacrifice myself temporarily to have it all.

One morning, four months after my third child was born, I woke up to the baby's cry and I couldn't move my right shoulder. It was red and hot. I ignored it and figured it was a trauma I couldn't remember. Three days later, my left fourth finger was red and hot. I started having trouble buttoning clothes. A day later, I felt like glass shards were piercing the bottoms of my feet.

I still ignored the pain. I started taking the elevator at work because my feet hurt too badly to climb the stairs and I couldn't bend my knees. After about a week, I knew that something was really wrong. I recall the day vividly, almost as if it was a dream.

The alarm went off at 5:30 a.m. I remember feeling exhausted in my bones. I could barely get out of bed. I hobbled down the stairs to let the dog out, but my feet were worse than ever. It seemed like glass kept cutting my feet. I made it downstairs, but I could barely open the door for the dog. Then the baby cried. I started to run up the stairs on impulse, so the other children wouldn't wake with the noise. But I couldn't run. Every bone in my body burned. I couldn't climb the stairs to reach her. I can still taste the salt in my mouth from tears as I had to crawl up the stairs. I remember reaching her crib but not being able to lift her out. It was then, as I lay on the floor crying so that my husband had to pick up the baby to give her to me, that I realized I was in real trouble.

Two weeks later, I had a diagnosis of severe rheumatoid arthritis (RA). My rheumatologist looked at my inflammatory markers and told me that my prognosis would be severe and debilitating if I didn't begin advanced therapy immediately. After my first meeting, I was fairly sure that I would no longer be able to practice cardiology. All the pictures from medical school of advanced RA came flooding back. The baby was now five months old, and I was nursing. My rheumatologist told me to stop nursing as soon as possible because he was very concerned about the destructive signs that my lab markers portended and about how symptomatic I was. He wanted me on drugs within one week.

So, I followed his advice. I took the drugs. I stopped nursing my baby. I cried every moment of those seven days. Every time I heard the baby cry, I had to walk away. My breasts were engorged and painful, yet I could not feed her. I want to cry as I write this because of the deep sorrow I felt at those moments.

I felt my choice was taken away from me; I had to give up something that was so dear to me. But every patient learns quickly that you have few choices. As patients, we rely so much on our physicians and suspend our own disbelief — even if we are physicians ourselves. I know I did.

As I started losing my hair and my daily nausea became more severe, I felt more and more bitter and lost. I started to blame my daughter. I thought that if I hadn't had a third child, none of this would have happened. After a few months of being on the medications, though, I started to feel better. I became better adjusted to the drugs and had fewer side effects.

It was around that time that I started coping with my disease, but I still hadn't released the anger. I still blamed my little girl for my disease. One day, about six months after beginning my treatment, I met a woman who would soon become a dear friend. She was a holistic nutrition consultant and was interested in educating my patients about diet. I was immediately skeptical, as are so many physicians about the role of diet. She offered to do my nutrition profile. That's when I started considering the effects of the foods we eat on inflammation in our body.

It is commonly thought that people develop illness after their bodies incur multiple "insults." The first insult is often genetic, then environmental triggers add to the initial insult. For instance, a person may be genetically predisposed to heart disease (the genetic insult) and has high LDL (bad cholesterol) and low HDL (good) cholesterol levels. Then, she adds a diet rich in saturated fats and hydrogenated oils, plus a sedentary lifestyle and perhaps smoking (the environmental insults) and we have a woman with heart disease. Similarly, with autoimmune disease, there is a genetic component, then we suffer some environmental insults that create stress (oxidative stress), which then triggers inflammation and leads to chronic illness.

Those environmental insults/triggers can be different things to different people—lack of sleep, cigarettes, excessive sun, saturated fats, gluten, dairy, animal food products, drugs (prescription or not). Understanding what causes the inflammation is the key. I, and others, believe that the foods we eat often trigger this inflammation. Many of us have found that simply changing the diet, cutting out inflammatory foods and adding back spices that decrease oxidative stress also lower the inflammation.

It takes time to learn our own bodies' sensitivities. Dairy and other animal products are often the source of inflammation. I was already vegetarian, so I started with dairy elimination. I cried when I gave up my pizza. Like most Americans, I also worried about not getting enough calcium and protein in my diet. It took me a lot of self-teaching to understand that so much of the calcium and protein we eat comes from the beans and greens we are eating.

The first few weeks of dairy elimination were very difficult. But since then, I haven't looked back. I have learned how to eat a plant-based diet with gusto. I enjoy kale smoothies in the morning or a bowl of oatmeal with cinnamon, beans and lentils for lunch and nuts for snacks. I eat chia seeds for their anti-inflammatory effects with my morning shake. I have salads with black beans and a teaspoon of turmeric mixed in. I marinate kale in hummus and don't use dressings that are full of oil. I have learned how to get protein from beans, calcium from greens and iron from black strap molasses and bean sprouts. I drink 64 ounces of water daily. I walk and walk. I sleep and I meditate.

It has been ten years since my diagnosis, but it took me four years to admit to others that I had an illness. I felt that if I said it out loud, people would judge me or think I was less adequate as a physician, as a mother and as a person. Now I realize it is *because* I have an illness that I understand and connect with my patients better. I can relate to their reluctance to take medication. I feel their fear as if it were my own. I feel their helplessness and anger as the fire in my own heart. I also know now that at the end of the day, we are all affected. Then, it is about learning to avoid environmental triggers and nurturing our bodies with a plant-based diet, low in oils and refined sugars and undergoing lifestyle changes such as increasing sleep and more vigorous activity.

It has taken me a long time to embrace my disease. I have learned that it is not illness that defines us but rather how we respond to it that makes us who we are. A person like me who was so controlled and rigid falls hard when illness hits. I blamed my daughter for being the cause of my illness. I was angry and mad for a long time, but now I feel healthier than ever before. My cholesterol is super low. I have no inflammatory markers, and I take no medications.

I feel great. I am strong. I ran my first triathlon. I have learned to take time for myself. I have learned to laugh more and not worry so much about being late or about climbing a ladder. I thank my body every day for what it has to give me, and I forgive it for what it cannot.

In some ways, the crazy thing is that getting sick was the best thing that happened to me. I have my girl to thank for bringing me back from a world in which I was drowning.

I realize now that my daughter didn't make me sick, she saved me.

Monica Aggarwal, M.D.

FROM DESPAIR TO DIGNITY
WILL IRVING

Conditions: Drug addiction, Alcoholism, Overweight, Depression, brain fog, PTSD

Will Irving's family had a cattle ranch. Meat was always on the table. As a teenager, he became an alcoholic and addicted to drugs and food. He became obese and depressed. He ended up in a juvenile facility. He was headed for death or prison. Today, Will has reversed his obesity, addictions, and depression through a whole plant food lifestyle. He does construction work for a gas utility. He's a blue-collar vegan. Will sees a big need for blue-collar people like himself to spread the word about plant-based nutrition to other blue-collar people. His story in this book is an important step in that direction. **@wgi61**

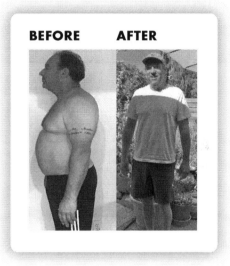

BEFORE   AFTER

At age 50, after 25 years of physical labor, my body was shot, along with key markers for my mental state.

My back, knees, neck, shoulder, you name it; hurt all the time with various degrees of pain. Also, my agility and balance had seemed to disappear over time. I found myself stumbling over my feet. Simple tasks, like putting up Christmas lights, became "scary" events.

How did I get here?

For what it's worth, my background is a bit unorthodox. My family background is in cattle ranching. We owned a cattle ranch. We had meat constantly.

Sexually abused at age 5, I had shut down emotionally at an early age. I suffered from anxiety and was afraid of the dark. People and new places were terrifying. At 17, I became incarcerated at Los Angeles Juvenile Hall. I was really terrified.

As a skinny white boy, I had zero "cred" and was an easy mark. I was definitely uncomfortable in the Juvenile Hall population. That changed somewhat when we were at the swimming pool one day. The guards started betting on who could beat who. I swam all through high school and was a competitive swimmer. I was beating everyone in the pool, slowly working my way through the lower ranked gang members up to the leaders of the *Bloods*, the *Crips*, and then the Hispanic gangs. Finally, a 30-year-old sheriff announced he was going to beat me in a 2-lap race. I beat him by a mile. The guys in Juvenile Hall loved it, and I got my "honor" by being the dude that beat the cop in the pool.

So, now I had my "cred," but I was still anxious and uncomfortable. My solution was to become heavily addicted to alcohol – it was a blissful escape. Drugs soon followed, and the cycle of heavy chemical dependency began.

At age 21, I began working in the construction trades, where I could hide out and develop a completely different persona than the basically sweet kid I really was. I worked first as a roofer, then as a carpenter. After that, I worked for a major utility company.

At age 26, I found myself to be the youngster in Alcoholics Anonymous (AA). I have stayed sober for 33 years now. But soon after joining AA, I found that much drama was to come, even sober. I gave up alcohol and addiction and chose food and people. Drama with people kept me far away from my feelings, and food kept me happy. Or so I thought. Both, however, turned out to be just as dangerous as alcohol ever was.

Food was a source of comfort and my reward during the day. A typical day included fast foods, chips, and diet soda by the liter. Breakfast was a gas station burrito, and a bear claw danish washed down with coffee or a Mountain Dew. Lunch was no better. Dinner was pizza, chips, burgers, fries and maybe a stray vegetable. I figured compared to drinking I was money ahead. Being young, I still seemed to be getting away with this crazy diet.

At 31, I suddenly went raw vegan. This began from reading every self-help book I could get my hands on. Working hard in my AA classes to be a kinder person, some of the books I read on self-care pointed to a vegetarian lifestyle as a better way to live, so I was going to change everything. For me, when I put animal welfare over my own desires, it has the natural effect of softening me at the edges. If I'm caring for an animal, I must also care about myself, in a kinder and softer way. With compassion and love.

Seriously, a year ago I would have gagged at writing this!

So, I became vegan. But my girlfriend at the time thought this was all very "girly." She wanted me to "eat like a man" because she thought that by avoiding plant food and eating more meat, it would make me even better in bed. So, being a good co-dependent, I ditched all the vegan stuff and went back to my previous eating patterns. I had been trending "nice guy," but she wanted "tougher guy." I obliged. We got married and had two daughters, in addition to the two boys she already had.

Slowly, I got heavier and more unhappy. Always feeling a bit depressed, I sunk even deeper into what would eventually become clinically depression. My muscles were getting soft, my stomach was getting bigger and bloated, like it was all inflamed with fat. My thinking was foggy and fuzzy. I was snoring and waking up, not able to breathe. My wife was getting mad at my shape and my moods, at my snoring and lack of interest in life. We got divorced.

Then, yoyo dieting began. I'd lose 20 pounds and gain it all back, lose 30 pounds and gain 30 back. Up and down with every fad diet and unhealthy supplements. As I got heavier, everything got worse. I was fat and depressed. My source of comfort was food, and more food. Pizza, chips, and Diet Pepsi. Dairy, beef, pork. Anything that was fatty and salty.

I was working late nights and eating fast food on the way home. By 11 pm, I had fueled my body with 2 to 4 energy drinks on top of 4 to 6 cups of black coffee. Heartburn was a nightly experience, and I began to wake up vomiting. That would be after eating a half carton of ice cream to "soothe" my stomach.

Now the eating was catching up to me. In short order, I was diagnosed first with high cholesterol, then with high blood pressure, and finally type 2 diabetes with an A1c level of 10.[1] and glucose at a steady 400. My weight hit 270, and very little of that was muscle. I had a brain wave scan and was off on every health marker. A diagnosis of sleep apnea soon followed, and I had to wear a CPAP machine and a mask that covered my face and nose just to be able to sleep.

So here I was again, killing myself. I didn't really care. Food was my pal, and I wasn't letting it go. Look, it wasn't alcohol, so leave me alone.

My daughter, Cynthia, who goes by "Max," was a hard-core vegan because of her love of animals. She kept dropping hints and suggestions, which I ignored or even ridiculed. She would label all my foods and how they affected the world ethically. She would tell me what alternatives were available. As a hunter and coming from a background of cattle ranching, I found this all to be just ridiculous. Meat was my way.

I was taking 3 medications just to break even. I had a machine I needed to use to help me breathe at night. I felt horrible. But I wouldn't give up my meat.

Then in 2018, I agreed to give up all animal products for my daughter – for one month. Almost just as a joke, but also to make her happy. I never looked back.

At first, I ate all vegan junk foods. All the comfort foods and processed stuff. My blood work was still bad.

In 2019, I saw a small vegan group on Facebook and joined. I just wanted to lose 20 pounds, but it ended up changing my entire life. With the support of my Facebook tribe, I started losing the pounds. I developed a new mindset, which allowed me for the first time to be more compassionate and kinder – first to others, and then myself.

As I started to like myself, I started to eat a whole food, plant-based diet. At first it was just for weight loss. Then I got my blood work back. It was much improved. After 6 more months, it was all normal. I was reversing what I had been told was genetic and not reversible. The chronic conditions were being healed by simply eating plant-based food, and doing moderate exercise, but mostly through diet.

HERE IS WHAT HAPPENED:

I went from 260 pounds to 195.
My cholesterol went from the upper 300's to 190.
My triglycerides went to a normal level.
My systolic blood pressure dropped from 170 to 100.
Blood glucose went from 200 with medication to 95 without medication.
I stopped snoring and no longer need a machine to sleep.
And my diabetes went from an A1c level of 10.1 to 5.2.

All of this was based on diet. No medications.

HERE IS ALSO WHAT HAPPENED:

My balance came back.
My confidence rose.
My pay at work went up 30%
Instead of sliding, I was thriving.

With my life experience, I should have been dead or in jail. Now I feel awesome. No aches, no mystery pains, no depression. I look 10 years younger.

All this from ditching all the BS preconceptions about what being vegan is all about. I have a new positive mind set – at age 59, I feel like life is just starting, not ending.

In short, plants saved my life in more ways than one.

Not bad for a former troubled teen, drug addict, alcoholic, ex-hunter, blue-collar worker that decided to give plants a chance!

After 28 years, my ex-wife wrote to me, out of the blue, to say how sorry she was that she didn't support me when I went vegan the first-time, years ago. She was sorry that she had "altered [my] path" because she wanted a tough, meat-eating guy in bed.

How glad I am to have come back to that path, though it took years, and a lot of pain and suffering, to get back to it.

Will Irving

---

[1] A normal A1c level is 5.6 or less. Pre-diabetes is defined as 5.7 – 6.9. A1c above 6.9 is diabetes. Normal fasting blood glucose is under 100.

FROM STROKES AND SURGERIES TO HEALTH AND INDEPENDENCE

JIM MCNAMARA'S STORY
AS TOLD BY HIS DAUGHTER, MOLLY MCNAMARA

Conditions: Cardiovascular disease, stroke, overweight

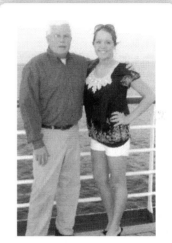

Jim McNamara & daughter, Molly McNamara

Jim McNamara grew up in the Midwest eating the typical American diet – burgers, fries, sausages, pizza, eggs, chicken, cheese and nary a vegetable. At age 55 he had a stroke. That started a series of stents and surgeries on several arteries in his body. Many surgeries and stents followed, but things just got worse and worse. The multiple surgeries and stents became a nightmare of useless but harrowing procedures. Fortunately, Jim met Dr. Caldwell Esselstyn, Jr., the author of the bestselling book, Prevent & Reverse Heart Disease. Note: Dr. Esselstyn wrote the Foreword to this book. Following Dr. Esselstyn's guidance to adopt a whole plant food lifestyle with minimal fats and oils, Jim experienced a stunning reversal in his health. Today, Jim speaks at Dr. Esselstyn's seminars for people with cardiovascular disease. He also has spoken on CNN and the BBC. Jim is a member of the Facebook group, Plant-based Cle.

He sat in a small, white-walled room, the sounds of doctors and nurses chattering outside the door. When the doctor walked in, Jim McNamara sat with his wife, Emer, and heard words he had already heard too many times, "The surgery failed."

It had been four years since the first surgery, with many surgeries to come. Lots of scars reminded him of past failures: On both sides of his neck, two more on each of his inner thighs, another one on his right calf, and a small one on the inside of his ankle.

It all started in March 2006. He had left the office early, telling his secretary that he didn't feel well. She responded, "You don't look so good." Jim arrived home and parked his car. Recalling that day, he said: "I remember feeling like my hands weren't working. My arms just felt as though they were rubber. Something was not right."

After a long day of feeling extremely fatigued and not himself, Jim decided to go to the emergency room. His wife left her office and met him there. As they waited for the doctor, Jim fiddled around with his left arm, trying to make a stiff fist with his hand, and said to his wife, "It's almost like I had a stroke." She refused to believe it, thinking, "There's no way it's a stroke. That can't be it!"

Within minutes, the doctor delivered the news. It was a stroke and they needed to admit him to the hospital right away. The news was a complete shock. Though the symptoms he had were all similar to the common symptoms of a stroke, Jim and his wife never seriously thought it could have been that.

Jim had a family history of heart disease. He had lost his dad to a heart attack when he was a teenager. "I can't blame everything on heredity, though," said Jim. "I did my fair share of unhealthy things for many, many years. And even though I gave a lot of them up a long time ago, sometimes the damage can't quite be undone."

The day after the news of the stroke, things seemed to take a turn for the worse, "I think he probably had another stroke in the middle of the night," said his wife, "because he seemed to lose the function of his left leg, too."

The doctor told them that the reason for the stroke was likely due to high blood pressure breaking off a piece of plaque in one of the two carotid arteries in his neck that supply blood to the brain. A plaque fragment traveling to the brain could cause a stroke. A 60 percent blockage in his right carotid artery needed to be surgically removed right away to prevent any further damage.

The surgery went well. Jim stayed in the hospital a few days, and then was able to go home. He arrived to a house full of party trays with meat sandwiches, cookies, a crock-pot of pot roast, and a pile of get-well cards. Two weeks of just sitting around passed, and then it was time for a follow up visit with the doctor.

Again, he was lying in a small, white-walled hospital room, waiting. The doctor's assistant did an ultrasound of his neck over the six-inch long scar from the surgery. The fresh scar was swollen with stitches. Jim was hoping and praying that everything would be okay, that the blockage would be all gone. The assistant said nothing, stared at the ultrasound results for a couple minutes, then left and returned with the doctor. The doctor looked at the results, then felt for a pulse in Jim's neck. He did not find any. The ultrasound did not show the carotid artery, either. The artery had occluded completely. It shut down. The entire artery seemed to have disappeared.

In a complete state of shock, disbelief and panic, Jim tried to get more answers from the doctor. How did this happen? Does this happen a lot? What do I do now? Questions raced through his mind. He wondered if he was going to die.

The doctor told Jim that this had never happened before. He had never heard of an artery completely occluding after this kind of surgery. The doctor explained that it was possible to live with just one carotid artery, but because that was the only one he had left, Jim would have to do whatever he could to keep it clear of any blockage. It was all he had left, and without it, he could not survive.

"I didn't have a crystal ball, I didn't know what might lay ahead, I just knew I had to take care of the one I had left," said Jim.

In March 2010, Jim walked from his house to the corner of the street to pick up his son from the bus stop. The walk was two minutes. He noticed a recurring pain in his left calf, as if the muscles were tightening together. "Even going into a store, my leg would cramp up," said Jim. "I couldn't walk any distance without pain."

After a couple weeks of hoping the pain would go away on its own, he decided he would get things checked out. Then, Jim started noticing a tingling sensation in the toes on his left foot when he was sleeping at night. He woke nearly every night with the tingling sensation coupled with a feeling of coldness in his foot. Jim knew it was a blood flow problem and it was only going to get worse.

Jim and his wife sat in a small, white-walled room again, only this time it was at the Cleveland Clinic. They had switched doctors, and now went in to see a highly recommended vascular specialist at the Cleveland Clinic. After describing the pain in his calf to the doctor, and after some tests, the doctor diagnosed Jim with peripheral artery disease (PAD). He explained this is a condition in which arteries in peripheral limbs are narrowed by a build-up of blockage thereby causing restricted blood flow.

Jim had a significant blockage in one of the arteries that brings blood flow through his leg and down to his foot. The solution to this was another surgery. The doctor assured Jim that this surgery was common, and they would put a stent in the artery. The doctor recommended a vascular surgeon.

"When I went in for surgery, I knew it wasn't as major as the previous one," said Jim. "It wasn't as invasive a surgery as the carotid was."

Later, Jim and his wife learned that the surgery was unsuccessful. It failed to adequately remedy the blockage. The doctor explained there was another surgery they could do — a bypass. They could take a vein from his right leg and put it into his left leg, creating a new passageway for the blood flow, bypassing the blockage. This surgery was more invasive. But there was one more roadblock before it could be done.

The doctor explained that Jim's left carotid artery, the only one remaining, would need to be cleaned out before they could go through with the leg bypass surgery. Because blood pressure fluctuates during any type of surgery, the doctor feared that if the carotid artery had too much blockage, not enough blood would make it to the brain during surgery. His one remaining carotid artery must be in the best shape it could be.

"I was scared to death to have it done," said Jim. "It was the only one I had left. I have only one chance. What's to prevent the same thing happening this time that happened before? That's when I thought this could be the end."

Finally, after about seven hours of surgery, they cleared out the blockage. It was a relief, but not completely. They still had another surgery ahead and had to hope this artery would not collapse like the first one. Two weeks later, it was time to head back to the Cleveland Clinic for an ultrasound of the carotid artery that had been cleaned.

The doctor said the first ultrasound did not look right. The tension was unbearable. The doctor did a second ultrasound. This time, the doctor said the results were much better and the surgery was fine. The carotid artery was clear enough to proceed with bypass surgery on his leg. The bypass surgery would leave him with an incision from his groin all the way down his left leg to just above the ankle, and another incision on his right leg from where they would take a vein to place in the left leg.

The surgery lasted hours, but when it was finished the doctor said he believed it was successful. A day later, however, there was another blockage and Jim had to go back into surgery to try and save the bypass. Jim finally thought he would stay in the hospital a few days, then go home and end this nightmare.

"I just was exhausted," Jim said. "It seemed like it was surgery after surgery, and I was ready for it to be over."

Jim stayed in the hospital for a week, and then was sent home. Four weeks passed, and it was time for another check-up. Jim went back to the Cleveland Clinic, back to a small, white-walled room to hear the latest news. The doctor took the ultrasound of his leg to check the blood flow after the bypass surgery.

"The bypass shut down," said the doctor. "It's not working anymore, it failed."

The doctor was direct, he did not try to sugarcoat the situation. After all the surgeries, all the hours spent in these small, white-walled rooms, after all the incisions made all over his body, it didn't matter. Jim sat covered in scars and finally felt defeated.

Jim said, "I just began to feel like my whole life was consumed by asking doctors what was next, what was the next step or surgery. It gets tiring, I never wanted to give up, ever, but I did kind of resign myself to this life. I figured I was going to have these issues all my life until it eventually killed me. There was nothing I could do."

The doctor echoed Jim's thoughts, saying there was nothing more that could be done. Jim would have to hope the blockage didn't worsen over time. Sitting in this all too familiar room, the moment was so surreal. After everything he had been through, it seemed there was no hope. No surgery could fix him, nothing could help. Everything was just a new scar, a new recovery, a new challenge. All these surgeries were supposed to make things better, but here he was feeling like they were all a waste. What could he do next?

In March 2011, his wife had heard of a radical diet created by Dr. Caldwell Esselstyn of the Cleveland Clinic, which was supposed to reverse and prevent heart disease. She researched both the diet and Dr. Esselstyn and found out that he was holding an all-day seminar in a few days.

With no other options left, Jim and his wife went to the seminar to learn about this diet. The diet seemed extreme, especially for a 100% Irish, meat-and-potatoes guy like Jim. The diet allowed only plant-based, whole foods, with no oil and minimal fats. Nothing that comes from an animal is allowed, meaning no meat, poultry or fish, and no dairy or eggs. Jim was skeptical he could ever do it, but knew he had no choice.

Jim recollected, "I never thought I'd be able to do it. My life was going to be terrible. I can't go out to eat. I can't eat normal food at my daughter's wedding. All these things went through my mind at the time. They were *meaningless* compared to what it has done for me."

After only 8 weeks on the diet, Jim went in for a check-up with his regular doctor. The results from the diet were immediate. In those 8 weeks, his total cholesterol dropped to 73 and his sugar level went from 104 to 89.

The next check-up was with the vascular surgeon who had done the bypass surgery and had told him there was nothing more he could do. This was 12 weeks into the diet. The doctor ran some tests, came back into the room and said, "You're my star patient! Have you been exercising?"

Jim explained he had not been exercising, but he was on this new diet. The 12-week results showed that the blood circulation to his foot had gone up from 47 percent to 63 percent, solely from the change in diet. His doctor was amazed. He had never seen such dramatic results before simply from a change in diet.

"As bad as I felt the day that doctors told me an artery had shut down, or a bypass stopped working – the lowest I had ever been – this was equally as great a feeling as when I saw the results from this diet," said Jim.

Dr. Esselstyn kept in frequent contact with Jim. And after each time Jim got blood work done, he called Dr. Esselstyn to report the results. After seven months on the diet, Jim walks through the park visibly slimmer, having lost about 30 pounds, and he is noticeably healthier. He only wishes he knew about the diet sooner. He could have prevented all of the surgeries that did nothing.

Each day he walks 45 minutes in the park near his house. It was only a year earlier that he could not walk more than 2 minutes without pain.

"The thing that gets me is why doctors don't tell patients about things like this diet before they go in and do surgery. Things are fixable without drugs and surgery. I feel compelled to get the word out that there's another option, and you don't have to go through what I went through," said Jim.

That small, white-walled room Jim has found himself in too many times hearing the words of failure from his doctor is no longer a place he dreads. He looks forward to the next time he can sit in that familiar room because he now knows he isn't waiting for bad news, or the next surgery option. He's waiting to hear how much of an improvement he has made.

"It's really a feeling of independence, because now I feel like I'm fixing myself. I'm not going to use surgery, I'm going to get better on my own," says Jim as he sits at the kitchen table with a giant plate of steamed vegetables in front of him and a smile on his face.

Molly McNamara

FROM MS TO HEALTHY MOTHERHOOD
MICHELLE O'DONOGHUE, M.D.

Conditions: Multiple Sclerosis, vision problems

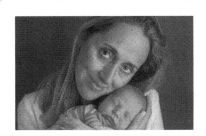

Dr. Michelle O'Donoghue & her newborn baby

Dr. Michelle O'Donoghue is an Associate Professor of Medicine at Harvard Medical School and a practicing cardiologist at Brigham and Women's Hospital in Boston. At age 33, she was diagnosed with multiple sclerosis (MS), with 25 lesions in her brain. Dr. O'Donoghue reversed her multiple sclerosis through conversion to a whole food, plant-based lifestyle. She is now a vocal plant-based diet advocate at her hospital, and at the American College of Cardiology Lifestyle and Nutrition Council.

I will never forget the moment that the neuro-ophthalmologist turned his back to me and announced to a group of medical students, "As you can see, this patient's brain MRI has all the classic findings of multiple sclerosis."

At that moment, I felt like the rug was being pulled out from under me and I broke down sobbing. Those words changed my life forever.

It was only a few days earlier than I had begun to lose vision in my right eye when I was returning from a medical conference. Over the course of two days, my vision loss rapidly progressed until I was completely blind in that eye. As a physician, the possibility that my symptoms could be explained by multiple sclerosis ("MS") had entered my mind, but I had promptly dismissed the idea as I had never previously faced any real threat of serious illness. After all, I was relatively young and living with the false shroud of invincibility that often exists in youth. "How could I possibly have MS?" I had asked myself. With those words, I moved into a phase of several months of denial as I evolved through stages of grief.

Fortunately, the possibility that diet may play a role in the progression of MS seemed immediately intuitive to me. If the body was inappropriately attacking itself in this autoimmune disease state, then it seemed probable that something was driving that confusion. I might be able to play a role in altering its course.

During my first meeting with the neurologist, I asked him if there might be a role for diet and he did not dismiss my question. Rather, he directed me toward a few studies that had examined diet patterns and progression of MS. He cautioned me that firm evidence was lacking, yet he had several patients who swore that adoption of a plant-based diet had made a positive impact on their symptoms and the course of disease.

During those first few months following my diagnosis, I read multiple books about MS that painted a very bleak picture and suggested an inevitable downhill course. I initially followed the path of more traditional medicine and started daily injections that were quickly upgraded to intravenous medication as my MRI showed further signs of progression. My follow-up scans revealed that I had more than 25 brain lesions, several of which appeared to be new and showed signs of active inflammation. During this time, I had convinced myself that adopting a whole food plant-based diet was simply too challenging, so I instead relished going out to restaurants to eat soft cheeses and meats with my friends as my disease insidiously continued to progress.

Like many people, I was under the delusion that my diet was already healthy because I was eating all the food groups "in moderation." To that end, I had been fortunate to never struggle with my weight and this had always given me the misguided impression that I could eat anything that I wanted. I assumed that having a normal weight was essentially a demonstration of health and therefore a "free pass" to eat as I desired.

In my youth, I was often teased for being underweight. So, in response, I often went out of my way to eat large fatty meals when I was around others because I didn't want anyone to walk away with the impression that I was "high maintenance" or a picky and selective eater. These bad habits slowly evolved, and I eventually found myself opening my drawer at work every day to raid a large stash of candy. Sure, I ate processed foods, but I never seriously considered how these might be slowly damaging my body and immune system.

I can't tell you exactly when something shifted inside me, and the light turned on. After several months, I walked back to my bookcase and re-read a book by Dr. George Jelinek called *Overcoming Multiple Sclerosis* that endorsed a primarily plant-based diet with lifestyle modifications. His book resonated with me as he himself was a physician who had a diagnosis of MS which had led him to carefully curate the evidence that concluded that dairy and meat were key drivers of MS progression.

Importantly, the idea that changes to my diet and lifestyle could ultimately alter my disease course was greatly empowering and gave me a renewed sense of hope. The next day, I woke up and adopted the changes overnight. It's now been more than 10 years since my diagnosis, and I'm overjoyed that I have yet to suffer a single clinical relapse and that my brain MRI has remained stable. Although I am eternally grateful for my physical health, I am even more appreciative of the lessons that a diagnosis of MS has taught me about myself during this unexpected journey.

We cardiologists often talk about the epidemic of obesity and the fact that negative lifestyle choices might be fueling diseases of the heart and blood vessels. However, we rarely have a serious discussion about the fact that positive diet choices may also be able to halt or even reverse disease progression. Certainly, the concept that diet may play a role in several disease states was never seriously addressed while I was in medical school.

Most physicians don't have either the time or training to sufficiently educate patients about diet choices. I recall routinely instructing patients to follow a "healthy diet," but that was the extent of the discussion. My own personal journey has opened my eyes to the powerful impact that a plant-based diet can have for allowing a person's body to begin to heal on its own.

A few years following my diagnosis, I met a loving man whom I later had the good fortune to marry. His support throughout this journey has been tremendous and unwavering. The first night we met, I shared with him my passion for better understanding the role of diet in disease and he immediately expressed a shared interest. Since my MS had been stable for several years and I wished to become pregnant, I made the decision with my neurologist to stop my MS medications. Several years later, we were blessed by the birth of our son who I delivered three weeks before my 44th birthday! Although the risk of MS relapse is known to be highest in the postpartum period, I am very fortunate that my health has remained stable, and I have better energy than I did when I was 30 years old. (This serves me well with a newborn!)

For anyone who is currently facing illness, I believe that adopting a plant-based diet can deliver a sense of hope and inspiration at a time in their lives when things may seem quite hopeless or overwhelming.

I never expected that facing my own diagnosis might make me a better physician. I have gained a deeper understanding of the role that diet, and lifestyle may play in so many different disease processes. In that sense, I truly believe that one has nothing to lose by embracing a whole food plant-based diet and adopting positive lifestyle modifications, as these changes can only lead to a place of greater physical and spiritual health.

Michelle O'Donoghue, M.D.

FROM CRISIS TO FREEDOM
ESTHER & BEN LOVERIDGE

Esther's Conditions: Obesity, depression, GERD, diverticulitis, bipolar, prediabetes, hypertension, sleep apnea, gastritis, pancreatitis, anemia, insomnia, vision problems, gallbladder disease, hyperlipidemia, constipation, hypothyroidism, knee problems

Ben's Conditions: Obesity, kidney stones, arthritis, appendicitis, ulcer, cellulitis, sleep apnea

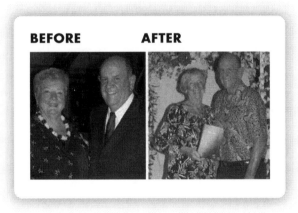

Esther Loveridge obtained a BA in Psychology from California State University. She met her husband, Ben, at his Baker Ben's Donut Shop, and they married and blended their two families from previous marriages. They worked and traveled together and ate out a lot. Eventually, Esther weighed over 280 pounds and suffered from a multitude of ailments, as did Ben. She discovered Dr. John McDougall's program for a whole food, plant-based lifestyle and her life changed dramatically. She changed her lifestyle and her health in her mid-70s. "It's never too late to get healthy," she tells everyone. Esther lost 130 pounds and all her ailments. Ben, who, at first, was resistant to the plant-based lifestyle, eventually came on board and lost 60 pounds and 20" from his waist. He also lost all his ailments. Esther has a highly popular Facebook group, "Esther's Nutritional Journey" where she inspires countless people to change their lives for the better. She has also published a book with her daily Facebook postings called, "From Donuts to Potatoes: My 366 Day Journey on a Plant Based Diet." Esther is active on social media encouraging people who want to follow and learn from her journey.

@estherloveridge

ESTHER'S STORY

We were at the end of our tour of beautiful, green Ireland in May of 2016 when I thought I just could not take another step. My knees and my feet were killing me as I inched my way to the departure gate at the airport for our trip back home. Ben, my husband, went on ahead of me and I felt stranded as I attempted to pull my own suitcase. Somehow, I had been able to keep up with our tour group, but now I just wanted to sit down in the middle of the terminal and "go on strike." I wanted to be saved and rescued. Giving up wasn't an option. Somehow, I mustered enough strength to do what seemed impossible and I made it to the gate on time.

I managed to recuperate after I got home. We even went to Universal Studios in Hollywood, California in June for our granddaughter's high school graduation party. I had lots of opportunities to stop and rest since I was too fat to go on some of the rides.

I didn't think I was going to die, but a funny aside is that Ben told me that I was going to have to write my own obituary because he just would not be able to write one if I died. One sleepless night, I got up and wrote it. I was only 72 years old and feeling okay, but two weeks later, my life completely turned around.

The big day came on July 13, 2016, when I had to face the prospect of an upcoming trip to China in September that would put me back on my feet for long periods of time. What was I going to do? I sought medical help and got some advice I did not want to hear.

I love having options in life. But this time, my options were limited. I was told I could continue taking pain medication, get injections in my almost bone on bone knees or be referred to an orthopedist for possible knee replacements. I didn't like any of those options, and I especially didn't like it when my doctor added "But, you'll have to lose 70 pounds before I can give you a referral."

That felt like a death sentence, or at least a prerequisite that seemed unattainable to me. I weighed 257 pounds (I was already down 25 pounds from my all-time high of 282) and had visions of someday getting down to 200 pounds. I was trying to be realistic, but 200 pounds was only 10 pounds higher than the 190-pound lie that had been on my driver's license for years. "70 pounds" echoed in my head as hopelessness enveloped me. He might as well have said I needed to run a marathon first.

How in the world could I lose 70 pounds? That really meant that I did not have any options, since I did not want knee injections, nor did I want to continue taking the pain medication on our next trip. Just in the nick of time, a good friend gave me a book which changed my life forever. She had been researching how to reverse diabetes. She came across the *McDougall Program for Maximum Weight Loss*, and she knew it would fit my personality and speak to me. I was a diehard dieter who liked to have results...fast. If weight loss was too slow, I'd give up again. This seemed to fit the bill.

I dove right into the material and quickly decided I would be my own guinea pig in this experiment with a plant-based diet. I almost angrily told myself, "I'm going to go 100% and put this guy, Dr. John McDougall, to the test and if I'm successful, I'll give him all of the credit!"

How was I to know that my need to lose weight would introduce me to a whole new world of living without eating animals or dairy products and ultimately reverse all of my other chronic diseases?

Sure, I had a long list of "ailments," but I never thought I was sick. I figured that I was healthy, even though my medical record listed me as being morbidly obese. Yes, I also dealt with other issues over time – GERD, diverticulitis, high blood pressure, high cholesterol, pre-diabetes, sleep apnea, low thyroid, gallbladder disease, pancreatitis, constipation and back spasms. But none of that mattered to me since my medications included statins, levothyroxine, sleeping pills, pain medication and lithium, all of which seemed to take care of me very well.

A new life emerged as I followed the plant-based diet very faithfully. We did take that trip to China in September, and it was amazing to me how quickly the diet acted as a toxin-reducing process in my body. The swelling in my knees was reduced by 4 inches!

At the onset of the diet, July 13, 2016, I took my measurements and set some goals: "I want to: Eat plant-based foods, lose 70 pounds, lower cholesterol, refrain from pain and sleeping pills, increase joint flexibility, lower blood pressure and improve my eyesight before July 13, 2017."

Now what made me think of my eyesight? I don't know. But as it turned out, that improvement also occurred. By July 13, 2017, one year later, I had lost 80 pounds and was well on my way to eliminating my medications. I learned that we could still travel and even take long cruises around the world while following our new diet. My knees were not going to limit us anymore. And they no longer needed to be replaced. I had renewed my lease on life.

We were on a cruise to Southeast Asia in 2017 when I had a discussion with the Tai Chi instructor about my weight loss. I was asked to share my good news with some of the students. That "talk" was videotaped and put on YouTube as *Esther Loveridge's Drastic Weight Loss Secret*.

Back home, at the gym, a water aerobics class student suggested I start a group on Facebook to share my success story. At first, I was hesitant but then I realized it might help others. I could clearly observe that water aerobics alone did not seem to be a way to lose weight. Additional opportunities to share my story came. Before long, I realized how much it would help to let others know that at 72 years of age, it was not too late to reverse all of my food borne diseases. I also wanted to give back to Dr. McDougall for saving my life. I decided to enroll in Dr. McDougall's *Starch Solution Certification Course*, which I passed in August 2018. That was a way of increasing my knowledge about a starch-based diet while also saying "thank you" to him and his program in a more meaningful way.

One by one, I was able to eliminate my medications. The last medication to go was the levothyroxine for my hypothyroidism. As my weight fell, so did the dosage of my medication from 112 mcg to 100 to 75 and finally down to 50 mcg. I was so close to a home run, and I wanted to be medication free. My doctor said if I were to eliminate the dosage entirely, I might regain some weight or have less energy. We agreed to give it a 6-week trial, after which I was retested. Happily, I continued to have lots of energy and my weight continued to fall. That last drug was eliminated in September 2018.

Another way of thanking Dr. McDougall was to attend his 3-day weekend seminar in Santa Rosa, CA in September 2018 where I got to meet him in person and have him autograph his "magic book," the *McDougall Program for Maximum Weight Loss.* My weight loss continued for a total of three years, until I lost not just 70 pounds, but 130 pounds.

Remember me wanting to improve my eyesight? Well, after just a few months on the diet, I saw my ophthalmologist who was following me for a macular pucker, pseudo-exfoliation and cataracts. He said I finally qualified for eye surgery. Hesitantly, I responded, "Well, I've just started a new plant-based way of eating and I kind of believe that it will help my eyes as well." He agreed that there was no hurry and he'd have me return for a checkup in six months.

With each successive visit, my eyes continued to improve until December 10, 2018, at which time I asked him if I should continue to wear my glasses to protect my eyes. His response was "With your eyesight, you don't even need to wear glasses." In October 2019, the Department of Motor Vehicles removed the corrective lens requirement on my driver's license.

On January 1, 2020, I made the decision to do another experiment. I wanted to learn to respond to my internal cues to decide when and what to eat. I no longer wanted to depend on an external device, like the bathroom scale. I had learned how to follow the guidelines on the calorie density chart which meant that I was eating fruit, vegetables, grains, and legumes. As long as I chose food from those four food groups, it didn't matter when, why and how much I ate. All that mattered was what I ate.

This concept made food choices so easy. I knew I had found the secret to never dieting again. No longer did I worry about the possibility of regaining any weight. I was home free. After 6 months, I checked it out. Not only had I not gained any weight, even during the Covid-19 virus time of isolation, I lost another 3 pounds and settled in at 127. After a full year of maintenance, I continued to wear a size 6 instead of a size 24-26!

It is not always easy living in a "mixed marriage," where we eat differently. At first, my husband Ben said, "I could never eat like you." I just replied, "OK."

Nine months later, after the last of the meat was out of the freezer and the cheese, mayonnaise and oil was out of the house, he joined the "team" and has since reached his goal. Ben's highest weight had been 322. When he switched to a whole food plant-based diet, he weighed 230 pounds. On this diet, he has reached his goal of 160 pounds on a 6-foot frame.

Ben thought he had been "fairly healthy" despite having bouts of cellulitis and kidney stones. He had arthritic pain in his knee and in his shoulder. After converting to a whole plant food diet, those are now gone, and he is totally medicine free. Ben no longer uses a sleep apnea machine. At his highest weight, his waist was 52 inches, but now he wears a 32" belt.

The clarity of mind, the stableness in my emotions, and my heightened spiritual journey have been rewards I never dreamed of just by switching my diet. Truly, all of my "ailments" are gone. Now at 77, I feel brand new.

Back on July 8, 2016, I was taking Zolpidem, a sleep medication. Ongoing health conditions were listed as Hypothyroidism, hypolipidemia, depression, diverticulosis of colon, anemia, iron deficiency, gastritis, pancreatitis, bipolar 1 disorder, insomnia, hypertension, prediabetes, and vitamin D deficiency.

In July 2021, just two years later, my doctor read off all these conditions to me and after each one, he said "gone" and removed them from my records. My July 1, 2019, summary reads "No medications marked as taking."

Let freedom ring!

Esther Lebeck Loveridge

BEN'S STORY

When I was young, I suffered from childhood obesity all through school. I was active in sports, and in high school I dieted and exercised. I got down to a normal weight. By the time I was 21 years old, I had bought two donut shops and again, the weight came back. After ten years, I went into business for myself and opened several Baker Ben's Donut Shops in the Sacramento, CA area. I continued in the donut business for about 20 years. It is amazing that I escaped type 2 diabetes since my father, mother and sister all had it. By working nights, I was able to further my interest in sports by coaching my daughters' softball and soccer teams. They never thought I worked!

I met my wife, Esther, in 1987 when she came into my shop as a customer. I hooked her putting a note in her donut bag! We got married 20 months later.

I sold the shops in 1988 and went into commercial real estate sales. In 1993, Esther took early retirement. We accepted positions as a sales team with a national marketing group. For several years, we traveled constantly on the road as sales reps, and we both enjoyed traveling in our territory in the Northeast. We did that for 30 weeks out of the year. A lot of traveling. We ate out 28 out of those 30 weeks. A nice big dinner was our reward to ourselves after a long, hard day.

I became obese, reaching a high of 320 pounds. All my life, I avoided going to the doctor because all he wanted to talk about was my need to lose weight. Around the year 2000, we went on a low carb diet and joined a gym. Over a number of years, I got down to the 220-230 range, but could not get any lower.

My wife, Esther, started the McDougall Maximum Weight Loss Program in July 2016. At that time, I said, "I can't eat that way." But I told her I would support her by not bringing any sweets into the house. I did most of the cooking, so I just continued to cook my own meals after that.

After several months of watching documentaries with Esther, listening to podcasts, and attending conferences with her, and seeing the results she was getting, I decided that when the meat in the freezer was gone, I'd give up meat. Next came the butter, cheese, eggs, and oil.

I actually never tried to lose weight on the plant-based diet. It just fell off. I continued riding a bike at the gym and within 6-12 months, I had gone from 220 to 160, which was just fine for my 6' frame.

I was fortunate that I had never been on medication for high blood pressure or anything. I did have sleep apnea and took Tylenol PM to help me go to sleep. I was hooked on it. Now I don't have sleep apnea and have no trouble going to sleep. Some of the health issues I have had over the years have been a few bouts with cellulitis, kidney stones, bleeding ulcer and ruptured appendix. Now I do not have those health issues and I do not require on-going medications.

My waist size has gone from 52" to 32," and my shirt size has gone from XXX large to a medium. I can now buy clothes anywhere. This is a new life!

I am also very happy that eating this way is helping the planet and the animals.

Ben Loveridge

FROM FAST-FOOD PHYSICIAN TO PLANT-BASED RUNNER

ALLAN KALMUS, DPM

Conditions: Obesity, hypertension, kidney disease, kidney stones, blood in urine, sleep apnea, joint problems, high cholesterol, prediabetes, asthma

Dr. Allan Kalmus is a podiatrist, and a foot and ankle surgeon in Michigan. He is a member of the teaching faculty at Beaumont Hospital in Wayne, Michigan. Dr. Kalmus was obese, adding 5 pounds of weight every year, and suffered from a host of issues. Like people everywhere, he relied on physicians and medications to treat his myriad problems. But they were never reversed and often got worse. After reading about the benefits of plant-based nutrition on the web, he decided to give that lifestyle a try.

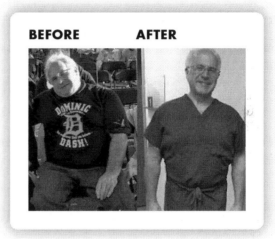

BEFORE   AFTER

He has never looked back. His only regret is that he did not start sooner.
Twitter: *@01newlyvegan.com*

In 2013, my blood pressure was 144/90, pulse 86 beats per minute, total cholesterol 234, and there were traces of blood in my urine under a microscope. I had 5 red blood cells per HPF (High Power Field). There shouldn't be anything in the urine other than, well, urine. My hemoglobin A1c level was 5.8%, which means pre-diabetes.

I had severe sleep apnea. I had a sleep study done that showed I would stop breathing over 600 times in an 8-hour period. I was not getting any quality sleep and felt tired all day. When I was driving, I was drowsy, catching myself nodding off at the wheel. I was prescribed a CPAP machine in 1999 to help me sleep. It was quite effective, and I felt much better.

My doctor gave me Lisinopril, an ACE inhibitor, for high blood pressure. It came down to 132/85, but my pulse stayed around 86 beats per minute. My elevated total cholesterol was treated with Simvastatin. It went down from 234 to 192. I was told that anything under 200 was healthy. I stayed on that for about 10 years even though my joints were achy. I knew about statin drugs causing severe muscle problems but did not know they also affect joints until

I was on them. When the pain got in my way, I would also take some aspirin, Advil, Aleve, or Tylenol.

The traces of blood in my urine had been there for more than 15 years. It never changed much until I developed a bad sore throat with a fever. The fever was gone in a day, but two days later I was peeing blood. I was sent to a kidney specialist who asked me if I had life insurance. I did.

The kidney doctor wanted to put me in the hospital and do a kidney biopsy but said he was not worried about any type of cancer. I asked what he thought it was? He spoke about the sore throat and how antibodies that formed may now be attacking my kidneys. My question was how would a biopsy change my treatment options? Would I need to take steroids or was there something else to do about it? He said "no." There was no treatment. I would either get better on my own or I would not, and my kidneys would fail. So, I saw no point in the biopsy and declined the test.

My kidneys got better on their own. I went back to having just 5 cells per High Power Field while eating the standard American diet "SAD" that I had always been eating. A few years later, a kidney stone happened. The pain was horrible. I was lucky and it passed on its own with the help of two pain pills, but the next day I was peeing blood again. After a week, it cleared up and I was now sent to a different kidney specialist. He did an ultrasound, which showed other kidney stones, but he said they were in a stable place and could be left alone.

He was more concerned with the chronic traces of blood in my urine. He told me I had "Thin Basement Membrane Syndrome." He put me on a second blood pressure pill to reduce stress on my kidneys. My blood pressure went down to 120/80 most of the time. It would range up to 130/85 and that was acceptable to my doctors. I continued doing what I normally did.

I showed up to my doctor appointments. I peed into the cup when asked and continued to spill an average of 5 red blood cells per High Power Field. I was also told to stop taking any non-steroidal anti-inflammatory drugs (NSAID) such as Motrin (Ibuprofen), Aleve (Naproxen), Indocin (Indomethacin), aspirin and others due to side effects that result in kidney dysfunction. The side effects are more common in people who have a history of kidney problems like mine, which may cause permanent damage.

My doctors were adding and subtracting pills, as they were trained to do. I was hooked up to a machine at night to keep me breathing. Aerobic exercise, especially in the cold weather, was out due to the asthma attacks it would bring about. Even without asthma, I had no desire to exercise at all. The only thing I did was what I referred to as "aerobic imaging." That means I would lie on the couch and imagine an activity.

During the summer I played a little golf once a week using a cart, which was really just standing around most of the time, and what I would call "swimming," or playing in the pool with the kids. My 10-speed bike was sitting unused, rusting in the garage with two flat tires that looked like they had suffered a moth attack. The tape on the handlebars was shredded. The bearings were even catching. Metaphorically, my bicycle and I were in the same shape.

Let's review; I was morbidly obese and pre-diabetic. I had high blood pressure, obstructive sleep apnea, high cholesterol, kidneys that leaked blood, kidney stones and aching joints. I was sedentary and had exercised induced asthma. Following any type of aerobic exercise, I would wheeze for hours. But, if you asked me how I was, I would tell you that I was feeling great, just fat.

This was all normal for me. Anything new that came up was just chalked up to normal aging. I didn't know any better. I asked my personal doctor what I should do to lose weight. He said, "You know what to do. Eat less and exercise more."

Obviously, I did NOT know what to do because every year I found myself to be at least five 5 pounds heavier than I was the year before.

Proper nutrition was of little interest to me. I would drive between offices and eat chicken nuggets, double cheeseburgers, and milkshakes. French fries were a big part of my lunch menu. Chicken, beef, milk, cheese, margarine or butter, fish, white bread, white rice, olive oil and eggs were my staples.

When I was younger, I used to think that I could exercise off any excess calorie intake. That, of course, never worked. Even when I was in college and was very active physically, the math just wouldn't come out in my favor. For example, going by the treadmill display, running one mile would burn off approximately 140 calories. According to McDonald's website, one double cheeseburger, large fries and a large soft drink contains 1230 calories. I would have to run 8.8 miles to burn off the equivalent number of calories. Eating approximately the same meal just three times a week means that I would have to run 26.4 miles every week to burn it off. That would mean running more than a marathon each week, just to burn up one lunch three times a week. Clearly, you can't beat a bad diet with exercise.

My focus at that time was to provide for my family. Between working, driving, and paperwork, my work week was 75-80 hours. As far as wellness was concerned my doctor was in charge of that. Maintaining my health was not something for me to control. I went to my doctor appointments and took my pills for blood pressure and cholesterol control. I felt fine. I had enough to worry about without adding concerns over my own health to the load. I was happy to delegate those worries to my doctor.

After all, there really was not anything I could do about it. My aunts and uncles with their various health issues were vanguards of my future genetic destiny. My mother, her two sisters and three brothers were a melting pot of medical issues. Their mother and father died from cancer and heart disease. Those problems were passed on to my mother's generation along with Type 2

Diabetes and Alzheimer's Disease. I trusted my doctor and advances in medical science to help me control any of those issues as they developed. Worrying about it wasn't going to change a thing.

But then, I finally made the changes I needed to do. After reading some of the good information put out on the web about preventative medicine and a plant-based lifestyle, I made up my mind to give it a try for a year. If I could improve my cholesterol numbers, lower my blood pressure and avoid heart surgery like my dad had at age 72, just by changing what I ate, there wasn't really any downside to it. So, I bought a vegan recipe book, picked up a few things like kale, quinoa, steel cut oats and nutritional yeast that I had not heard of before.

I started cooking. I began to run, cycle and swim. I started a blog. I developed recipes and posted them to keep myself going and to connect with others.

Nobody changes until they are ready. Change comes from within. The "Zen" of change, from the within to the without, may come from a variety of precipitating factors.

TO THE READER: IF YOU ARE AMONG THOSE WHO REQUIRE A SCARE, READ ON.

Heart disease is the #1 killer in the United States. If you are waiting for a diagnosis, consider the fact that 50% of first heart attacks are fatal. Autopsies have shown that children who die from a variety of unrelated causes, such as car accidents, already have fatty streaks in their hearts and arteries. *(Journal of Clinical Nutrition).* In other words, stop thinking about waiting to take care of your heart until after you develop symptoms. The disease is already there, and the first symptom is, half the time, sudden death. There is strong scientific evidence that reversal of heart disease is consistently achievable through diet.

You may be mindful of a gradual increase in your weight over the years. Diabetes may be on your mind. In most cases, intramyocellular lipid accumulation, the fat buildup in the liver and muscle cells that comes with obesity, is the underlying cause of insulin resistance, leading to adult onset (Type 2) diabetes. The longer you wait to start taking care of yourself the harder it becomes to avoid heart disease, kidney failure, blindness, uncontrollable infections, and amputations related to diabetes. It is a downward spiral despite the best medications and the dietary guidelines of the *American Diabetes Association.*

There is a far superior approach to controlling diabetes. It is safe, effective, cheap, available without a prescription and already in your hands. It is available at every grocery store, everywhere. If I can do this, you can do this.

AN UPDATE DURING COVID-19

As much as I hate to admit it, without actually making me sick, COVID-19 and the pandemic have taken a toll on me.

Before Covid-19, I was as close to the whole foods, plant-based lifestyle, with no processed oils, as I could get. Running, bicycling, swimming and weight training at the gym were all part of my normal routine. My food was void of any animal products and I wasn't eating any processed or packaged foods except for whole wheat or gluten free pasta. Occasionally, I would break the rules and have some chips at a party or share some veggie straws with my grandsons, but for the most part, I was compliant with the WFPB-NO lifestyle.

The virus came and the stress level went way, way up. I had far less business than normal. It was scary just going to the grocery store. Walking outside downwind of another person could be risky, even when wearing a mask and gloves. We didn't know if breathing within 10 feet of another person or even touching an elevator button and then your own face would make you sick. The pool I would normally use for laps never opened last summer and the gym was shut down. I missed meeting my friends in the local plant-based community and going to the lectures.

I am a stress eater. With nothing to do but watch TV, or go in the kitchen and cook, I cooked – a lot! My cooking was completely compliant with no animal products and no processed sugar or oil, but my portion sizes and eating frequency both increased. I would sneak more chips and eat children's breakfast cereal when I got bored or stressed out. I gained back 15 of the 110 pounds I had lost and kept off during the previous 6 years. I could feel the difference in my clothes and felt flabby.

Every single day I would plan on putting on my running shoes and getting back out there, being stricter with my eating habits and limiting my portion sizes. So far, I haven't done a thing to help myself get back to my healthy habits, but I've come up with a plan.

Ironically, it's the same plan that got me started on this path but with a few minor tweaks to adjust for the times in which we find ourselves living.

WHAT I DO

- Keep an accurate food log. Write down the time and everything that is included in anything I eat. That means if it's oatmeal with cinnamon, turmeric, black pepper, strawberries, a banana and blueberries, write it all down including the water or plant-based milk used to make it. It's time to reconnect the brain with the stomach and be accountable for what I eat.

- Before eating, I read the last entry in my food log and decide if I'm just stressed and bored or if I'm truly hungry or thirsty.

Same idea: engage the brain before opening the mouth.

- When the urge to eat gets the best of me, I have healthy alternatives ready and waiting. Fresh vegetables and fresh fruit are easy to have handy just in case. Be accountable and write it in the log. Nobody joins Weight Watchers or other weight loss organizations because they ate too many apples and carrots.

- Together, we can do this. We all can get a little more exercise than we did the day before. I take the stairs. I walk. I jump up and down when I'm pumping gas. So can you. Park farther away from wherever you are going. Take an extra lap or two around the office. You can do this too! Wave arms in the air like you just don't care! Just do something to get your heart rate up a little more than the day before until you can work your way back to your pre-pandemic or pre reading this book level of activity... and write it in your log!

- Since gathering in large groups may change on and off, get engaged with the WFPB-NO online and experience this community again. Share your problems and your recipes. There is no shortage of online groups with whom you can interact. Look on Facebook for local groups like PBNSG. org here in the Detroit area or join the national Forks Over Knives Official-Plant Based Group. There are so many choices. Get involved with several that suit you best.

Try hard not to screw up, but when you do, forgive yourself and go back to step #1. No one is going to do this for you, but you can definitely do this for yourself! Your doctor is not in charge of your health. You are.

This isn't a diet, it's a lifestyle. Like most things in life, it's a journey and not a destination. Twists, turns, and bumps in the road add to the challenge and to the enjoyment.

If you're new to this, watch the movie *Forks Over Knives'*. It's still available on the free app *TUBI*. It's a game changer.

While you're at it, watch *THE GAME CHANGERS*!

And watch, *Eating You Alive* on Amazon or iTunes, or better yet, at www. EatingYouAlive.com. It's powerful and amazing.

There are a bunch of other great documentaries that will pop up on Netflix, but we all must start somewhere. If you have specific questions about carbs, protein, macro and micronutrients or how best to fight diabetes, high blood pressure, heart disease, etc. you can get them answered with reliable, science backed references by going to Nutritionfacts.org and plugging your question into the search bar. Michael Greger, M.D., has thousands of videos already recorded and transcripts of each one with journal references to help you.

For simple whole food, plant based recipes with no oil, I like PBNSG.org, since I occasionally contribute recipes. It doesn't cost much to join, but you can click past the sign-up page if you choose. My recipes are included at https://01reluctantvegan.blogspot.com

This really works and if you stick with whole foods, avoid the packaged vegan foods and read labels, not only will your health and weight improve, but you'll also save lots of money! WIN, WIN, WIN!!!

Collect a few recipes and get started!

"Accept the things you cannot change, change the things you can, and be wise enough to know the difference."

A parable revisited: One evening, an old Cherokee Indian told his grandson about a battle that goes on inside people. He said, "My son, the battle is between two wolves inside us all. One is Evil. It is ignorance, ego, greed, disease, and denial of truth. The other is Good. It is wisdom, joy, peace, humility, benevolence, empathy, compassion and truth."

The grandson thought about it for a minute and then asked his grandfather, "Which wolf wins?"

The old Cherokee simply replied, "The one you feed."

There is great wisdom in that little story. YOU are the one you feed. You choose every day the direction of your health and wellbeing. Either you will make the choice to feed your health, or you will deny the science and feed disease. It is that clear and simple.

Once you accept this brilliant truth a new and exciting pathway opens. No longer is ignorance your excuse. The seed has been planted, the path is open and your journey to health begins.

It is with every mouthful, that you choose which wolf you will feed.

Allan Kalmus, DPM

FROM TERMINAL CANCER TO FULL TIME WORK

DAN AND SHEANNE MOSKALUK

Dan's Conditions: Kidney cancer, liver disease, overweight, PTSD

Sheanne's Conditions: Obesity, depression

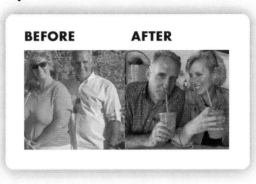

BEFORE   **AFTER**

Dan Moskaluk, a "Mountie" with the Royal Canadian Mounted Police, was diagnosed with terminal renal (kidney) cancer. His kidney was surgically removed, but the cancer had spread to lymph nodes and other critical areas of his body. He was told he only had a few months to live – two years at the most. Previously, Dan had been an occasional vegan because Sheanne, his wife, had adopted a whole food, plant-based lifestyle to lose weight and be healthier. Dan was not fully committed, but Sheanne, who had ballooned to 293 pounds, lost 133 pounds. Then, when Dan faced his terminal cancer, he was "all in." The oncologists told him he would get progressively worse, but he actually got progressively better. Months later, there was no longer any detectable cancer in his body. After two years, the outside date for being alive, he went back to work full time. Dan and Sheanne Moskaluk are now known as Indian Rock Vegans and are avid presenters of the plant-based lifestyle at healthcare conferences, podcasts and in the film, Eating You Alive. *Sheanne is certified in Plant-based Nutrition with e-Cornell, and both are directors with the Okanagan Health Forum.*

Facebook Group: *Indian Rock Vegans* | **Instagram:** *Indian Rock Vegans*

Our names are Dan and Sheanne Moskaluk. We are known as Indian Rock Vegans on our social media platforms. We live at Indian Rock, in Naramata, British Columbia, Canada. We both have experienced changes in our lives that we never would have believed possible. *We started by changing our minds and the rest followed.*

SHEANNE'S STORY

In 2010, our 14-year-old son became interested in weightlifting and bodybuilding. He joined a local gym, where he was told he would never gain muscle if he did not consume protein powders and lots of meat. So, being what I thought was a good mother, off to the local health food store I went. What happened next would drastically change our lives. While I was browsing the selection of whey protein, a salesclerk inquired if I was buying this for myself. I explained it was for my son, to which she quickly replied, "You need to do some research before giving that to your kids."

Well, that was unexpected! I didn't purchase any but instead, went home to Google whey protein powders. That's when I first stumbled across Dr. John McDougall in a YouTube lecture titled *The Perils of Dairy*. Honestly, I initially thought Dr. McDougall was some crazy quack, but I continued to listen. I watched the lecture three more times. The information he was discussing was completely foreign to me and the exact opposite of everything I'd ever been taught, but for some inexplicable reason, I was deeply intrigued.

Upon further investigation, I came across other doctors discussing the health risks of consuming meat and dairy. These doctors, Neal Barnard, T. Colin Campbell, Michael Greger, Dean Ornish, Hans Diehl, and John McDougall, led me down the rabbit hole to a parallel universe. As I read more over the next few months, it became abundantly clear that I could no longer feed myself and my family in the way I had been doing.

On April 1, 2011, April Fool's Day, after "leaning" in for a few months, I fully committed to a vegan diet. I cleaned out every cupboard, the fridge and freezer of any animal products and processed junk foods and started preparing exclusively vegan meals. At that point in time, I weighed 293 pounds. My story was common. I gained weight with the first pregnancy, then more with the second baby. I had tried every fad diet; Weight Watchers, Jenny Craig, etc., losing some weight and then gaining it back, plus more. At 47, I had resigned myself to the fact that I would spend the rest of my life being obese.

I had been a baker in a local coffee shop, using all my grandmother's recipes. If the recipe didn't have butter or lard, I wouldn't make it! Food was my currency. If someone did me a favor, I baked them a "thank you" cheesecake.

However, losing weight was not my goal when I adopted this way of eating because I had simply given up trying. I was more focused on avoiding the diseases that are so heavily linked to the consumption of animal products: heart disease, cancer, diabetes, etc., and protecting the health of my family. But to my surprise, that first month, I lost 15 pounds without even trying! That was with no exercise at all, because at nearly 300 lbs. exercise had not been part of my life. Cutting the lawn and vacuuming the house was exhausting!

Over the next two years, everything changed. I continued to educate myself by reading books, listening to webinars, and generally being obsessed with the topic of plant-based nutrition. I refined our diet from vegan to a whole food plant-based lifestyle, focusing on "food as grown" and reducing or eliminating many processed, packaged vegan foods and oil.

To the astonishment of my friends and family and myself, I lost a total of 133 pounds. It's hard to put into words the emotions involved in losing that much weight. It's such a struggle that seems unattainable to so many.

On more than one occasion, I would bump into someone who hadn't seen me since my weight loss and they would break down in tears, partly because they were happy for me, but largely because they never thought it was possible for themselves and I was living proof that it was. Several encounters with friends were downright awkward, as many didn't recognize me. If I was wearing sunglasses, they assumed that Dan had a new girlfriend. That is, until I spoke. Then their jaws would drop! Fitting back into my wedding dress, so many years later, was an overwhelming moment that I never imagined could happen.

I gradually added walking into my daily life. I now easily walk 5 km of very hilly terrain every morning. I had never gone to the gym, just hill climbing walks. My family was also on board with adopting a whole food plant-based lifestyle at home. But out of the house, they were still consuming animal products and junk food.

My husband, Dan, increased his health by lowering his cholesterol. He lost some 35 pounds and reversed metabolic syndrome symptoms and pre-diabetes, though he was not totally committed to a whole food, plant-based lifestyle.

As we approached being empty nesters and our retirement, we thought our health was bullet proof as we were both healthier than we had been in years.

DAN'S STORY

By 2013, Sheanne and I had settled nicely into our new lifestyle and were feeling great, until the week of November 9th. I had been experiencing increasingly severe abdominal pain all that week and after a day of splitting firewood, I could no longer ignore the pain. This culminated in a trip to the emergency room.

I was given a CT scan. Since kidney stones had run in my family, I was expecting the results of the scan to confirm my suspicions. With the scan results clutched in one hand, the doctor escorted us into a private room, and in two sentences the doctor changed our world. He stated, "It's not kidney stones, Dan, it's cancer. Your right kidney is one massive tumor, and it has metastasized."

The doctor added more devastating words. "You probably have no more than two years of life." I suggest you get your affairs in order and live those remaining months as well as you can."

His words still resonate in my head. Time was suspended as I processed what I had just heard. We would later learn more details — that it was metastatic Stage IV renal cell carcinoma, with the tumor having metastasized into the vena cava and throughout my lymph nodes.

As anyone who has gone through this will tell you, it truly is like having the rug pulled out from under you. Shock and disbelief were soon followed by devastation and grief.

It was at that very moment in the hospital emergency room, that I committed to fully adopting a whole food, plant-based lifestyle, 100%.

Why? Because I didn't want to die.

That week was spent advising family, friends, and coworkers. I took an extended leave of absence, something that I had never done during my career as a police officer with the Royal Canadian Mounted Police.

The prognosis was grim. In the immediate days following, we had been told by the specialist/urologist that I had only months to live, up to two years at most, and that it would be a miserable two years. We learned that kidney cancer is normally asymptomatic and often discovered by accident, and that a cancer of this magnitude could have been quietly growing for 10 to 15 years.

During those first weeks after the diagnosis, we felt like a couple that now had a third person always present with us. A heavy presence always just there.

I was immediately scheduled for a major surgery to have the kidney and surrounding lymph nodes removed. The tumor was also growing up the vena cava, the biggest vein in the body that carries blood back to the heart, The cancer was growing towards my lungs and heart. There was a chance that, since they would need to clamp off and possibly dissect a section of the vena cava, I could bleed out during surgery. So, my family and I spent our Christmas 2013 at the Vancouver General Hospital, wondering if it would be my last Christmas. Despite the cancer diagnosis, as grim as it was, my medical team remarked numerous times that I was extremely healthy and that I was an excellent candidate for the surgery itself.

On Christmas Eve, with a cardiologist on hand, two surgeons worked to remove my kidney. They successfully pulled the tumor out from the vena cava and removed several surrounding lymph nodes. They closed me up with over 50 staples across my abdomen. Earlier scans had shown that there were affected distant lymph nodes which could not be removed and would be monitored.

The surgery was a success and I remained in the hospital for 6 days. I don't recall very much from the entire hospital stay and surgery. However, one vivid memory sticks with me to this day. Following surgery, as I lay in my hospital bed, I glanced up at the large blackened tv screen that hung above my bed, and it reflected my image on the blackened screen. I had an intravenous line attached to my neck, one in my arm, an epidural needle in my back, oxygen lines in my nose and a catheter in my penis. I was shocked at what I saw, thinking to myself that never in my wildest dreams did I ever think I would ever find myself in this position. Yet there I was.

The oncologist had been clear in stating that, "We would be naive to think that the cancer would not spread and grow." We prepared for the worst.

At this same time, Sheanne had turned her attention to researching the effects of nutrition on cancer. We were shocked to find that there is 100 years of data linking animal foods to cancer cell growth, which further prompted her to continue with our whole food, plant-based lifestyle. Sheanne embarked on what she called our "program of nutritional excellence" focusing on tons of greens, beans and nuts and seeds, purifying our diet even more to a "cleaner" whole food plant based one.

The initial weeks following surgery were extremely difficult and I didn't think I was going to survive. I could not sleep nor eat due to the surgery, and the long list of medications that were prescribed for post-op recovery. With 50 staples across my stomach, suffering from insomnia and feeling nauseous, the nights were painful and often spent literally wringing out my empty stomach hunched over the toilet bowl. This brought a quick end to the prescription meds, as I thought I'd rather put up with a bit of pain rather than not sleep or eat.

I lost a drastic amount of weight and muscle mass, dropping around 35 lbs. As I regained my appetite, Sheanne thought that having me nibble freshly roasted raw nuts would be the easiest and best way to get calories and nutrients into me during that period of not being able to eat.

Slowly but surely, I recovered from the surgery and regained my strength. Knowing that I had to start moving, I used the treadmill in my bedroom, putting in 30 to 60 seconds a couple times per day at a very slow crawl. Just putting one foot in front of the other. I was eventually able to walk down the stairs to spend time in the living room, and later to walk up and down our driveway.

It was during this time that Sheanne received a phone call with the pathology results of the tumor tissue samples taken during surgery. She was told that they were very sorry to inform us that this was a very aggressive form of cancer. As Sheanne hung up the phone, she said to herself, "Well, that's it. I guess we're done."

What we've come to realize now, is that the petri dish provided a hospitable environment for the cancer cells to grow. However, in my body, we had created an inhospitable environment, thanks to a whole food, plant-based diet.

My slow and steady recovery provided us with hope. I never felt anger about my situation and essentially woke up each morning, opened my eyes and thought, "Okay, here goes another day."

I lived that day for the moment. Then, when I retired to bed at night, tucked in and closed my eyes, I thought about the day I had just lived and fell asleep. And then repeated this again and again. We had good days and bad days, filled with as much laughter as there were tears. We never realized how many tears the human body could make!

I'd always been a mindful person. As a police officer, I had been frequently exposed to human suffering and encountered many who's lot in life was worse than mine. This was especially so after completing peacekeeping duties with the United Nations in Haiti. As an operational police officer, meditation and the survival mindset were something that I practiced throughout my personal and professional life. Their importance was magnified, and their effectiveness amplified as a result of my cancer. As anyone diagnosed with cancer can attest, it can be a reawakening, bringing on a more intense level of mindfulness.

We are fortunate to live in the beautiful Okanagan Valley of British Columbia, overlooking Okanagan Lake. With my increased mindfulness, I spent a lot of time simply taking in the beautiful sights, sounds and smells of our rural home, after the household went to bed and before everyone woke up. As spring ushered in, I relished every moment.

It struck me as odd that my physicians told me that I would get progressively sicker and that my health would deteriorate, but here I was each day, feeling a deeper sense of growing wellness, as the weeks turned into months. My scans were showing no spread or growth of the cancer, which itself brought us more hope. Because of my excellent general health, terminal cancer aside, the oncologists felt that we could watch and wait as I healed from surgery, something that is not afforded to many cancer patients.

The doctors were amazed at my progress and remarked at how well the surgery site healed. Due to my overall good health, and the fact there are no effective treatments available for renal cell carcinoma, I was told that my best chance was to go into a Phase I drug trial for a new type of immunotherapy medication. I was accepted into the study. It was an immunotherapy protocol that consisted of four double drug treatments every three weeks, followed by a single drug treatment every two weeks for the rest of my life, or as the oncologist stated, for as long as my body could take it.

We were told that immune therapies boost your own immune system to attack the cancer. But it was a little like "letting the tiger out of the cage," and that it could attack any healthy organ by mistake. And attack it did. The tiger turned on my liver in a near fatal attack after only three treatments.

I was immediately dismissed from the trial study. It is hard to get a drug to market when it kills trial study patients.

Much to the surprise of my doctors, again I quickly recovered from the liver attack, with no permanent damage to my liver. Six months after the initial diagnosis of Stage IV terminal cancer, I was off all medical treatment. I continued to receive CT scans to monitor the cancer's progress, but to everyone's surprise, from the day of diagnosis onward, there was still no further spread of the cancer. The affected lymph nodes had started to shrink.

Stage IV renal cell carcinoma has a five-year survival rate for men of 5%. Ten months after diagnosis, the word remission was being used, and by February of 2015, the cancer clinic closed my file, stating that my cancer was radiologically undetectable.

At the two-year mark, when it was predicted I would die, I went back to work. full time. I continued not only to survive, but to thrive! My medical team referred to me as Superman, often remarking that I was an anomaly.

I am not an anomaly. I eat whole foods, plant-based. That's it.

We walked out of the cancer clinic relieved and feeling elated. We felt as though we had just won the lottery of my life.

While we are thankful for the medical support that we have through our healthcare system in Canada, we had disappointments. The most disappointing aspect of my treatment and care was that my oncologists and specialists showed no interest or curiosity in learning more about our whole food, plant-based lifestyle. It was something that they chose to ignore, with one oncologist criticizing us for speaking publicly about the benefits of this lifestyle, saying we were irresponsibly promoting false hope. We were deeply disappointed.

As a result of surviving Stage IV cancer and once fully recovered, I revisited another health issue, which as a police officer I had not fully come to terms with. That was seeking counselling for post-traumatic stress disorder (PTSD). This led to a formal diagnosis during my recovery period. Once again, upon further research on the health benefits of a whole food, plant-based diet, we learned about the role that it can play in helping PTSD and other mental health issues such as depression.

While still emotionally fragile, we were elated. We had weathered the storm and had come out the other side, but we could never have predicted what would come next. After seeing the trailers for a film titled *Eating You Alive*[1] one Sunday afternoon, Dan reached out to the co-producer, Merrilee Jacobs, to inquire about the release date of the film. Dan explained that the subject was dear to our hearts and briefly described how a whole food, plant-based lifestyle had impacted us both. One thing led to another, and by Thursday, we were travelling to Chattanooga, Tennessee, to have our story filmed. It was the first time that we had discussed cancer with anyone other than close family and friends. It was an emotional and exhausting day, but the thought that our story could inspire others and help people was exhilarating.

That exhilaration has sparked a deep desire in both of us to help others. *Eating You Alive* has given us a platform and the courage to springboard into advocating the benefits of a whole food, plant-based lifestyle. We are so honored and proud to be associated with this documentary; we view our story as a gift to be shared with others.

We now have many speaking engagements, both in person and on podcasts. Sheanne also co-facilitates the CHIP (Complete Health Improvement Program) that was developed at Loma Linda Medical Center. She has been doing this for the last two years, an experience she absolutely loves. The program runs three nights a week in Penticton, BC, for five weeks, and educates people about science-based benefits of adopting a whole food, plant-based lifestyle.

We are such different people now, viewing the world through very different eyes and all because of the simple change in what we eat. A whole food, plant-based lifestyle is the best diet for weight loss, which also happens to be the best diet for cancer, heart disease, diabetes, and many other chronic diseases. You don't heal just one thing; you heal the whole body.

Dan "I often state that it is because of Sheanne's beautiful intelligence that I am still alive today."

P.S. Our son never did take any protein powders. He gained tons of muscle and is committed to the whole food, plant-based lifestyle to this day.

P.P.S. In 2021, Dan celebrated his 8th year of cancer-free life after his diagnosis, and Sheanne has maintained her weight loss.

Sheanne and Dan Moskaluk, Indian Rock Vegans

---

[1] Purjes, the co-author of this book, is the Executive Producer of the film, *Eating You Alive.* The film is owned and supported by the Purjes Foundation, www.PurjesFoundation.org

FROM HEART DISEASE DISASTER TO PBNSG

PAUL CHATLIN

Conditions: Cardiovascular disease, angina, leaky heart valves, enlarged heart, heart murmur, overweight

Lying on a hospital gurney, Paul Chatlin was told by his cardiologist that he needed bypass heart surgery. His only other option was to try whole food, plant-based nutrition. He chose the latter and his life was radically changed for the better. He reversed several severe cardiac problems and was so energized and grateful for his renewed life that he started the Plant-based Nutrition Support Group (PBNSG) in his Michigan hometown. The group has now grown to many thousands of members with chapters in other communities. Paul invites everyone to join PBNSG wherever they may be and help spread the word.

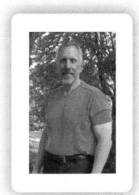

Website: *www.pbnsg.org*
Also on Facebook, Instagram, Pinterest *and* **Twitter.**

My name is Paul Chatlin. I was born in Detroit, Michigan and have lived in West Bloomfield, Michigan since 1971. I am in my 60s and married with several children and grandchildren.

My dad and all three of his brothers had bypass surgery in their 50's. Two never made it through the surgery, and one was never the same person again. My father cried in pain for four days after his bypass surgery. It was the only time I ever saw tears in my father's eyes. My local doctor said that the disease was in my genes. That was years ago. Today, I have never felt better! I was given a miracle.

I have three sons. When I was given the choice of bypass surgery to treat my own heart disease, or a nutritional change, I made the jump the next day to a whole food, plant-based lifestyle. My motivation for this lifestyle change was my love for my sons, and out of respect and love for my father and three uncles.

In May of 2013, I was diagnosed with heart disease. One artery was 100% blocked and two others were 65% blocked. Add to that leaky heart valves and an enlarged heart, thickening of the right side of my heart, a left bundle-branch block and a heart murmur, and I was in seriously bad shape.

I could not walk more than a few steps without excruciating pain in my chest. Doctors were not sure if I needed bypass surgery or a heart transplant. I was taken to the catheterization room at the Cleveland Clinic. There, a catheter was snaked up from an incision in my wrist to the coronary arteries in my heart. Contrast dye was then injected through the catheter into my coronary arteries so that blockages would be visible on video monitors. This allowed the doctors to assess my condition and decide what should be done further.

After the heart catheterization procedure, I was told that a heart transplant was not needed, but I did need open heart bypass surgery. Lying on the wheeled hospital gurney, I kept praying that this was not happening to me! I promised that if I could find a way to not have this surgery I would give back to others. I called it my "gurney promise."

As I was being wheeled toward surgery, my cardiologist gave me another option instead of bypass surgery: "plant-based nutrition." When I said I would try anything other than bypass surgery, he took his cell phone out and called Dr. Caldwell Esselstyn, Jr., the author of *Prevent & Reverse Heart Disease.* Dr. Esselstyn picked up the phone at 11:00 P.M. to take my doctor's call and talk to him. I did not know that Dr. Esselstyn had been his mentor in medical school. I was handed the phone and heard Dr. Esselstyn say, "Go on home, and I will call you in the morning."

That was it ... no open-heart surgery for me that day. I wanted to hear what Dr. Esselstyn had to say. As I look back, I realized that this was the first time I was connected with Dr. Esselstyn and my cardiologist together. I knew very little about nutrition and never heard anything about a whole food, plant-based (WFPB) diet. This was quite a leap of faith!

At 8:00 A.M. the next morning, Dr. Esselstyn called me and spoke to me for an hour. Thus began my plant-based nutrition transition.

After just three weeks, my angina disappeared! My cholesterol levels dropped from 347 to 127 in just one year. Today, it is at an amazing level of 92. Also, I lost 65 pounds, and have kept it off. I feel great!

Last year my wife and I paid almost $24,000 in medical insurance, yet we only spent $188 in medical bills for the whole year. Why? WFPB!

This whole food, plant-based lifestyle has saved my life.

I was given three miracles. (1) Getting into the Cleveland Clinic in just 3 weeks. (2) Being assigned to a doctor (it could have been any one of so many other doctors) whose mentor was Dr. Caldwell Esselstyn, the physician who wrote the bestseller, *Prevent and Reverse Heart Disease.* (3) Having Dr. Esselstyn pick up the phone so late that night, leading me to avoid having open heart bypass surgery.

IT WAS TIME TO GIVE BACK!

I attended a Plant Based Cooking Class hosted by Dr. Esselstyn and his wife, Ann. I was not a cook and did not have a clue about this lifestyle change.

I needed guidance. The cost was $975. I tried to have Blue Cross/Blue Shield reimburse me but was denied.

So, I thought, this is what I can do to give back. For three months I worked on Blue Cross/Blue Shield with no progress. After escalating the matter to the highest level, I was still denied because they did not have a pay code assigned for plant-based matters. They suggested I work with the state legislature for any hope of future change! I kept saying to them that I was amazed they would rather cut a check for $125,000 for bypass surgery rather than reimburse me for a cooking class for $975 to learn how to cook healthy, plant-based meals and insure I never need to have bypass surgery.

Right then, I knew the system was broken and I needed a bigger voice. Right then, the Plant Based Nutrition Support Group (PBNSG) was born. Today, it has thousands of members, with chapters in several cities around the country.

But I was still not well. My doctor told me I needed 60 - 90 days of bed rest to help shrink my enlarged heart and he believed this would stop my valves from leaking. During my bed rest, depression started to creep in. I am a positive person and a dreamer, so depression and negative thoughts were very new to me. I felt as though I was all alone!

I decided to put a small ad in the local paper inviting anyone who was interested to hear my story, see my cupboards, share my recipes, and be connected to me. The ad said something like this:
"I would like to share my experience with any person in our community who may be considering a nutritional change before pills or procedures. Who should consider this type of nutritional change? Any person who has had bypass surgery and hopes that a change in eating habits may prevent additional surgery. Any person who is in need of bypass surgery but would like to change their diet to whole foods, plant-based in hopes of not needing surgery (like me). Any person whose family has a history of heart disease and wishes to alter their current diet to possibly avoid health issues down the road."

In just two days, more than 20 people contacted me and I invited them to my house. What a wonderful evening we had! Some of these wonderful people are still PBNSG members today.

Each person who attended felt just like me. Alone, but hopeful. I ran the ad again the following month. Another 20 people attended. This led to the thought that I must start a whole food, plant-based support group to help others. I contacted the chief of cardiology at three hospitals in my area. I asked them to give me three names of cardiologists who might be interested in educating our community on the benefits of WFPB nutrition. Each of the three cardiology chiefs gave me the names of three cardiologists, but Dr. Joel Kahn was the only one that was listed by all three cardiology chiefs. So, I called him, and we met. It was "like at first sight." That day, Dr. Kahn agreed to assist me on this journey.

In February of 2014, we held our first Plant-Based Nutrition Support Group (PBNSG) meeting. I thought that having 20 - 40 people attend would be a great showing. But, amazingly, 123 people attended! And 23 people signed up as volunteers. The meeting was held at Beaumont Hospital in Royal Oak, Michigan.

The following month, in March, we held our second meeting. I thought there would be a significant drop in participants, but I was wrong. We had over 143 people attend! What was interesting is that of the 143 people, 44 of them were new faces. This meant that many more people were interested in reclaiming their health and that new friendships were being made.

In April and then again in May, we continued to grow. That growth has continued steadily, month after month after month. Today, we have almost 10,000 members and over 100 volunteers. Our web page is www.pbnsg.org and we have a presence on Facebook, Instagram, Pinterest and Twitter.

In addition, we started various outreach programs. One of them is our Medical Course Material, which we presented to the Wayne State University Medical School. The authors were first- and second-year medical students from several Michigan medical schools. This information is available on request.

Four local doctors offered to teach any doctor, nurse, or health professional the benefits of a whole foods, plant-based diet. The results were remarkable. 73 doctors attended, with 35 on the waiting list. There should be a program like this in every city and state!

Though no one can go backward and start over, anyone can start now and make a brand-new ending.

Paul Chatlin

FROM PANIC ATTACKS TO PLANT-BASED PEACE

ERIN & DUSTY STANCZYK

Conditions: Obesity, GERD, anxiety, panic attacks, hormonal imbalance, depression, brain fog, yeast infections

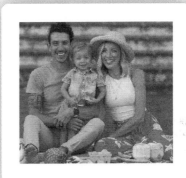

Erin and Dusty Stanczyk are certified health and lifestyle coaches and the creators of the lifestyle brand, www.EatMoveRest.com. They inspire others to get back to basics by doing 3 things we all do every day – eat, move, and rest. It all started in college when they were struggling with weight gain, anxiety, depression, and a plethora of health symptoms. They stumbled on a plant-based diet and spent many hours researching it in books, videos, and conferences. The whole plant food lifestyle has resolved all their issues, and they now work actively to spread the message to others. You can find the plant-powered family blending and chopping on **Instagram,** *@ErinStanczyk @DBStanczyk @EatMoveRest and on the* **EatMoveRest YouTube channel**.

AS TOLD BY ERIN

As high school athletes and straight A students, we were both brought up in healthy households, but by the time we got to college, we both derailed. For me, I was living off beef jerky and ramen noodles in my dorm room, staying out late, drinking, partying, eating fast food, sleeping in, and quitting all exercise.

I had begun to gain a significant amount of weight and began experiencing my first bouts of anxiety, depression, and debilitating panic attacks. My grades suffered, and I no longer felt like I knew which direction I was headed in life.

All of this was coupled with a series of inexplicable and disheartening health symptoms—numbness, tingling, brain fog, weakness, low energy, poor digestion, irregular cycles, constant yeast infections, acne, and severely interrupted sleep due to shortness of breath and tightness in my chest. I turned to "Dr. Google" (which quickly became my best friend and worst enemy). Everything I searched came back with terrifying diagnoses and prognoses, but I couldn't stop digging every time a new symptom or struggle came my way. I was thoroughly convinced that I had multiple sclerosis or some other sort of scary autoimmune disease occurring in my body. Every symptom seemed to fit the bill, and my heart sank. My anxiety and despair became even worse, and I began to obsess and fear for my future.

Coming from a family of doctors, my father being one, I was easily able to seek medical advice. Soon, I was visiting specialists for MRIs, CT scans, a nerve conduction study, and too many blood draws. There were no lesions on my brain, thankfully. But physicians and therapists couldn't give me a diagnosis or drug to "fix" my problems, as I was hoping, so I was left at a loss. It felt as if everything I was describing to every health professional was disregarded and chalked up to being "generalized anxiety disorder." I felt unheard, neglected, and a bit cheated.

Yes, I was anxious, but mostly because my life felt out of control. I didn't have a support system or solutions that would help me regain a sense of control over my unraveling mental and physical health. Even though I hadn't been given a labeled disorder or disease, I was still very much in a state of "dis-ease." Because I was also not getting regular periods, I was prescribed hormonal birth control to regulate my hormonal "mood swings," anxiety, and cycles.

Towards the end of college, my now husband, Dusty, and I lived together, and he was able to witness my nightly panic attacks, breathing issues, and the other symptoms that I was experiencing. He felt for me and was willing to do anything to help me get better. We began by getting active together—riding road bikes long distances, going for runs, and lifting weights at the gym.

Exercise only felt like a temporary solution for the stress and anxiety I was feeling. It was a momentary escape and release. Afterwards, though, I would still have to come home and lay down at night with the same symptoms and fears. We began cooking at home together more often, and went out less and less, but we were still eating the standard American diet (SAD diet). Unfortunately, in my attempts to lose the weight I had gained, I began counting calories, living on low calorie, processed Lean Cuisines and overexercising. I began to look emaciated. I lost weight (too much in hindsight) and was undernourished by the wrong foods.

I can recall at the time that a typical day of eating would look something like this: Religiously drinking powdered "meal replacement shakes" and eating scrambled eggs and hash browns for breakfast, cold cut sandwiches loaded with lunch meat and cheese for lunch, and grilled meat for dinner. Snacks were always anything that claimed to contain fiber on the packaging, from cereals to bars to yogurts, because my digestion was extremely slow, and I was bloated.

I would allow myself one piece of fruit per day, for fear it would make me "fat." I considered the leaf of lettuce and slice of tomato on my sandwich to be my vegetables for the day. Meanwhile, the ambitious, oversized bag of leafy greens I'd purchase weekly at the grocery store, would sit and wilt in the refrigerator until I'd throw it out and replace it again.

I hit rock bottom, so to speak, when Dusty and I were headed to San Diego for a quick vacation, and all of my symptoms came rushing in at once—

numbness, tingling, brain fog, muscle weakness, and panic. The flight attendants were unable to administer anything to me, and the flight was landed 30 minutes earlier than scheduled to be sent to the hospital by ambulance.

My blood was drawn. I sat and waited for hours. No red flags, no answers. Just a suitcase full of "natural supplements" that I had gathered thinking that would help "fix" me. I was prescribed Xanax, which got me through our vacation in a cloud — I was no longer anxious, just numb and deeply saddened. We made it through, but I knew I couldn't live my life continuing to just get by and get through. I kicked the anxiety meds and hormonal birth control, as well as my bag full of snake oil pills and potions.

Then, we were invited by my uncle, a cardiologist, to listen to a doctor at a local hospital speak on preventing and reversing heart disease through diet. That person ended up being Dr. Caldwell B. Esselstyn. We tried his food, we saw his charts, and we were so intrigued that we went home and immediately watched the documentary, *Forks Over Knives*. We weren't sure about taking the plunge into going completely vegan, so we started out going vegetarian for 40 days for Lent, along with my uncle and other family members.

After that, we felt amazing...and more importantly, we were just surprised and amazed that we didn't die from the "lack of protein!" We saw the challenge as completed and rewarded ourselves by going to our favorite drive-thru to celebrate with burgers and fries. We couldn't un-learn what we now knew, though, and we kept asking ourselves if it was worth it? We decided we'd try to continue a vegetarian diet. To replace meat, though, we were living on scrambled eggs, milk, Greek yogurt, and cheese to make sure we were "getting enough protein."

I come from a family with a history of heart disease, from a grandpa who's undergone several heart bypass surgeries, to an uncle who passed away in his 40s from a heart attack. Cholesterol and blood pressure medication is considered standard for most of my family members. As we became more invested in our health, we began routinely getting our blood work done. As a young 20-something, I expected everything to be perfect, especially after going vegetarian and doing daily workouts.

My dad's nurses told me my cholesterol levels had been trending upward, and it would probably be a good idea to get on a statin drug to keep things in check. When I asked for how long, the response, "forever," just didn't sit well with me.

Meanwhile, Dusty was struggling with severe acid reflux that would impact his mood, his sleep, and the enjoyment of any meal. It seems as if eliminating "trigger foods" like chocolate, red sauce, and other acidic foods didn't make a difference. The digestive tract simply wasn't healing. He was on multiple acid reflux prescription medications, and he was told to drink milk with his meals to neutralize the acid.

We began to revisit Dr. Google. This time, rather than searching for symptoms, we searched for natural solutions. We watched more documentaries, read more books, went to conferences, and found some inspiring people just like us who were all promoting a plant-based diet.

We decided there might be something to it, but the only way to find out how good we could truly feel was to go all-in on a whole food, plant-based diet. We weren't the cold-turkey type, but we continued, slowly eliminating dairy and then finally eggs, after which, my "hereditary" high cholesterol numbers dropped in a matter of weeks, to what Dr. Greger would call the "heart-attack-proof" range. Also seeing our inflammation (CRP) numbers change for the better, while also maintaining healthy B12, D3, protein and iron levels was all the convincing we needed.

The kicker for me was when my mental health improved drastically. No more unmanageable anxiety, no more shortness of breath, no more pins and needles, numbness, or tingling. There was less stress, and no feelings of depression or despair. And my panic attacks completely disappeared, allowing me to socialize again and sleep through the night.

It was a challenge to trust that we were getting what we needed without animal products, and we were constantly reading and researching websites such as **www.ForksOverKnives.com** and **www.NutritionFacts.org** for articles on protein, B12, Omega-3s, D3, and more. We were also thriving on the "Forks Over Knives" recipe app, which helped us develop a handful of staple recipes we loved that replaced our SAD favorites. The next hurdle for us was wrapping our heads around how we could cook and get enough fat without oils.

As soon as we began eliminating oils from our cooking, two things happened; my digestion became the best it's ever been, and Dusty's nagging acid reflux and digestive woes subsided over time as his gut healed. He can now enjoy his favorite Lentil Bolognese without any sort of flareup! So many of our preconceived notions and cemented beliefs in our minds had been busted, but each one came with its own struggle that we gave ourselves grace to navigate slowly and steadily. We attribute this approach to our long-term success, as we now come upon 7 years as whole foods, plant-based vegans.

Another major challenge for me was to trust that I could eat a lot of carbs and not have to worry about counting calories or restricting my diet and stay at a healthy weight. However, I tried it. I incorporated lots of delicious raw fruits and veggies and hearty cooked meals at dinnertime and was able to get more toned and muscular in the gym, putting on some healthy weight, and feeling the most comfortable I've ever been in my body and in my heart. It was once again just a reminder not to knock something until you rock it!

Our extended family and friends were highly skeptical at first, and probably assumed what we were doing was just a phase, a fad, or a trend. Over the course of the next couple of years, though, friends from high school and college began asking for "that green smoothie recipe," or what to do about their rising cholesterol or weight gain.

About two years into our success as fully plant-based eaters, we started our online business. We traveled to a series of health and lifestyle coaching certification courses around the country and began a website and blog to accompany our journey. That's how *EatMoveRest* was born. Eventually, the blogging and daily inspirational Instagram updates turned into a YouTube channel that has grown to over 112,000 subscribers! We'd hosted local and international retreats with amazing individuals from all walks of life, and we feel that this diet most certainly has become a lifestyle for us in every sense of the word.

We'd get comments from online followers and some family members that it's okay for a couple of carefree 20-somethings, but when you're ready to have kids, you'll have to go back. Quite the opposite happened. After being on hormonal birth control for 8 years, a lot of healing needed to take place. A healthy diet without a fear of carbs and calories, and free from animal products and processed foods, allowed my cycles to regulate on their own.

We wanted to be as natural as possible, and to our surprise and delight, we were expecting our first child in April of 2018. Now, I'd be lying if I said that I wasn't nervous yet again about whether this plant-based thing would work or not. While I had seen many vegan mamas on YouTube, I also felt it was important to seek out reputable sources and information from professionals.

The internet has done more good than harm for us, as Midwesterners. We are landlocked in the beef-eating state of Nebraska, so turning to social media has allowed us to find a community of like-minded individuals, as well as inspiring researchers, physicians, and nutritionists. We've come to realize that this plant-based lifestyle is a grassroots movement that requires a bit of homework on the part of the individual, because much of this invaluable information still hasn't hit the mainstream.

After educating ourselves, we now know that a *well-planned* vegan diet is healthful for all stages of life—including pregnancy, breastfeeding, and beyond.

We now have a healthy and happy plant-based 2-year-old, and baby number two is on the way. Confidence in any lifestyle change is key, but that confidence doesn't come without commitment. We committed to the journey, we educated ourselves, and we held fast to our beliefs and avoided nay-sayers.

It is so rewarding now, to be able to bring dishes to extended family gatherings, and see our family clean their plates. It is so meaningful now to go to our parents' houses and have them prepare their favorite plant-based dishes for us. It is so exciting now for us to see our younger siblings moving in this direction.

The support from friends and family isn't always there from the start, but the longer you stick with it, the more the interest, and eventually respect, will follow. We continue to lead by example, rather than preach, push, and prod, and those who come along for the ride never regret it!

Erin Stanczyk

GIFTED WITH THE DISEASE OF MULTIPLE SCLEROSIS

MARCY MADRID

Conditions: Multiple Sclerosis, vision problems

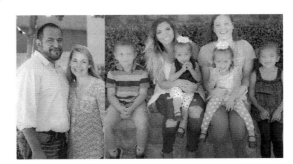

Marcy Madrid & family

When she received a diagnosis of a debilitating and incurable disease at the hospital where she worked, Marcy Madrid never would have considered that to be a gift, but that is what it turned out to be. When she was told she had multiple sclerosis (MS), Marcy's life came to an abrupt halt. She had lesions in her brain and was immediately put on cancer chemotherapy drugs. Those drugs are the standard treatment for MS and many other autoimmune diseases, because chemotherapy drugs suppress the immune system. She suffered hair loss, nausea, and other terrible side effects of those drugs. But not long afterwards, she went on a plant-based diet, stopped taking all the MS medications, and was amazed at how rapidly her disease reversed. It reversed so much that the lesions in her brain and spinal cord had all but disappeared. Find Marcy on TedX, and YouTube.

Well, that's odd, I thought. That annoying numbness that I felt after having my twins through a C-section started coming back. I know the doctors said it was normal to be numb for months or even years after a Caesarian, but I don't remember hearing it could go away and come back. Apparently, it was not normal. After calling my ob/gyn team, they suggested I see a neurologist. That's when the journey began.

At first, I didn't think much of it. I assumed they were going to tell me I had some nerve damage that could easily be fixed by doing x, y and z. I was young, healthy and at the prime in my life, with so many incredible things ahead of me to accomplish. The surfacing of a serious health issue never even passed my mind. I was totally oblivious, and I was really surprised when the doctor ordered an MRI. As my husband and I went back to meet the doctor for the follow-up visit, we braced ourselves for what was appearing to be a much bigger deal than what we had anticipated.

It was.

According to the physician, who had years of experience in reading these types of scans, it was the early stages of MS, multiple sclerosis.

OK, I thought to myself. I'm not going to lose it in the doctor's office. After all, this hospital was where I worked. These were my peers. This wasn't some private appointment; this was my professional setting. I needed to be strong and fully understand what he was saying, and what I needed to do next, before going to my next meeting. I remember my eyes tearing up as he began explaining the lifestyle changes, I may experience, but I choked back the tears with all my strength. This wasn't the time, nor the place. So, we wrapped up and I went on about my day.

For the next two weeks, as more information came out, as more doctors' appointments were made, as treatment regimens were discussed, that strength slowly began to unravel. I quickly found out that when you don't allow yourself to cry and let out all the emotions that naturally begin to build up after something like this, they will just creep up on you when least expected. You can't control it. Driving in my car, working in my office, using the restroom, lying in bed at night. These were all moments that I found myself bursting into tears, sobbing at times and desperately trying to pull myself together before someone found out. I had to stay strong before someone noticed my weakness peeking through the cracks.

Finally, I hit my knees in prayer and just wept. I had to completely surrender to whatever this was. I didn't understand it, but I was trying not to question. My mind became a battlefield those next few days. The letters M and S seemed to be playing on a continuous loop on a movie screen in my head. My thoughts were consumed with how I was now so different from everyone else.

Meanwhile, things seemed to be getting worse for me physically. I began MS medications immediately due to my doctor visits. I was told I had to begin these meds quickly to try and slow down the progression of the disease as much as possible. The hope was to delay the inevitable debilitation and wheelchair in my future.

MS is an autoimmune disease, where your own immune system attacks the nerves, tissues, and organs of your body. The conventional treatment for most autoimmune diseases is chemotherapy drugs, like the ones given to cancer patients. They weaken the immune system, so it lessens its attacks on the body. But they also have severe side effects, the side effects we hear about with cancer chemotherapy. And with a weaker immune system, there's a greater chance of getting some other disease.

Once I began taking the meds, the symptoms of numbness began to slowly fade away, but they were now replaced with hair loss, extreme fatigue, blurry vision, nausea, and tremors. And a whole new feeling of being sick. Now, for the first time, I actually felt like I had a disease.

My husband saw our lives change dramatically as I would be driven home from work by a coworker, unable to drive myself, and then collapse on the couch at 6:00 pm with no energy left to function or to care for our four young kids.

At this time, I was being introduced to research studies that had been done with plant-based nutrition as a treatment for MS and other chronic diseases. As my husband and I explored this information, we felt drawn more and more towards this approach for my own healing journey. After about a month of debilitating symptoms and harsh drugs, we felt I should stop taking all meds, and begin to treat this disease with plants. The MRI that diagnosed my MS disease took place in October of 2015. I went fully plant based and off all meds in November of 2015.

It wasn't easy. I cried all the way through the Thanksgiving holidays, as I faced the most intense feelings of social isolation, despair, and physical withdrawal. When I brought my early, tasteless plant-based experiments to my family's Thanksgiving dinner I became depressed. I didn't realize how hard it was to be different until then.

I gained confidence in knowing that being different isn't a bad thing when the common culture in our country is jumping off a cliff regarding health and wellness. I pushed on as I discovered a whole new way to cook and eat, and new foods to prepare that I didn't even know existed. As time went on, it got easier and easier. Eating plant based not only became my new normal, but delicious and enjoyable! I realized my taste buds and cooking skills just needed some time to adapt and catch up.

Along the way, my symptoms began to resolve themselves. My energy and vision returned, and I began to feel "normal" again. As I continued pursuing the food-as-medicine approach, I also awakened to a renewed purpose and a perspective of gratitude and faith in my life. This brought me a sense of peace and joy during this difficult journey we were facing.

I believe this is where the idea of lifestyle medicine came into play in my recovery and ultimate disease reversal. Not only did I change the food I was consuming, but I also had an improved and healthier mental, emotional, and spiritual outlook in my life. This did wonders for the continually stressed and all-consuming lifestyle I had been living. No longer did I wear stress and busyness as my badge of honor; now, I rejoiced in the importance of good health, and spending time with loved ones.

My neurologist admitted he did not know how to handle my case without meds, so he referred me to an MS specialist at UT Southwestern Medical Center in Dallas. Six months later, I had a follow-up MRI in April of 2016. When my husband and I went to the follow-up visit with my new neurologist, he was impressed to say the least. He put my MRI from October and April side by side and pulled us close to the screen. He pointed out a significant lesion on my brain in October that had all but disappeared by April. Noting that he never saw this type of regression, he was even more interested in my case, and how I was using food as medicine to treat this relentless disease.

Since that initial evidence of how food and lifestyle had reversed my MS, my health and quality of life have continued to improve. It hasn't been a perfect journey and I still struggle off and on with temptations to backslide in my nutritional choices or re-engage stressors in my life.

The beauty of my journey has been the growth and strength I've experienced in my soul along the way. Not to mention the transition to a healthier life that my husband and family have made in the process.

When I was first diagnosed in 2015, I thought my life was changed forever and I would never be the same. I was right, but not for the depressing reasons I expected.

Instead, my life is so much richer and fuller -- full of life and purpose, more than it ever was. The ordeal of MS turned out to be a gift of grace, a gift of a road to health, wholeness, and healing.

Marcy Madrid

GOODBYE LUPUS

BROOKE GOLDNER, M.D.

Conditions: Lupus, kidney disease, anticardiolipin disease, migraines, overweight

Dr. Brooke Goldner is a board-certified physician and bestselling author of the books Goodbye Lupus, Goodbye Autoimmune Disease, and Green Smoothie Recipes to Kickstart Your Health & Healing. She is a frequent speaker at healthcare conferences and has been featured in health magazines, podcasts, TV programs and films such as Eating You Alive. *She has guided hundreds of people to better health and disease reversal through her Hyper-Nourishing Protocol for Reversing Autoimmune Disease and through her website, www.GoodbyeLupus.com. She has published research in the* International Journal of Disease Reversal & Prevention *www.ijdrp.org on reversal of chronic kidney disease and is a regular contributor to the* T. Colin Campbell Center for Nutritional Studies.

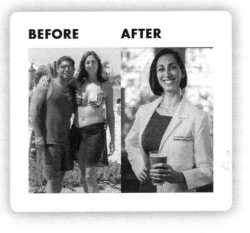

BEFORE   AFTER

Websites: **www.veganmedicaldoctor.com** & **www.goodbyelupus.com**

When I was 16 years old, my doctor told me I had six months left to live.

I was diagnosed with systemic lupus erythematosus and lupus nephritis. I was in stage IV kidney failure. It was so severe that my doctor told me that the best-case scenario with standard treatments was dialysis; the worst-case scenario was death.

For a couple years before this diagnosis, I struggled with severe arthritis and debilitating migraines, but it was a rash that made me go to the hospital. It was a butterfly rash, going from one cheek to another. My parents and I suspected something was wrong but we had no idea the diagnosis would be so dire.

I was positive on every test for lupus. My ANA was positive (indicating that my immune system was attacking my body), my DSDNA lupus antibodies were over 2,000, and there were massive amounts of proteinuria in my urine. The subsequent renal biopsy showed stage IV membranoproliferative nephritis type 2, an advanced form of the most aggressive lupus-related kidney disease.

Treatments at the time were mostly steroids and similar medications, which my nephrologist told my family would not be sufficient to save my kidneys. He talked to us about using Cytoxan chemotherapy to shut down the autoimmune disease. At the time, chemotherapy was an experimental treatment, but now it is standard. He explained that chemotherapy suppresses the immune system, and since lupus is an autoimmune disorder, they thought suppressing the immune system would help. In a sense it worked. I went into remission by having chemotherapy for two years straight, once a month.

I was simultaneously taking 60mg of prednisone a day as well as Premarin and Provera to protect my reproductive system, calcium carbonate to try to counteract the bone loss from the steroids, an ace inhibitor for renal protection, antiemetics for side effects of chemotherapy and others as needed.

It was a difficult, painful time. I would spend a week vomiting after each chemotherapy treatment and was afraid to eat during that time. As the weeks passed, I would slowly build up strength, and by the time I felt more normal, I was due for the next Cytoxan treatment, at a stronger dose than the previous month. My family was amazingly supportive and helped me get through.

I was still in high school. I focused on what I could do. I didn't know how much time I had left on the planet, so I wanted to make my time matter. I wanted to help the health of others and reduce suffering. My passion was for science, so I decided to become a doctor. I took any moment I felt well to read ahead in my textbooks, since I never knew when I would be too sick to participate in class.

I got a scholarship to my dream school, Carnegie Mellon University. It was an incredible time, as my first day of college was one week after my last chemo treatment. I was in remission during college. Every test was still positive for lupus, but I was stable, and my kidneys were no longer failing. I still had to be careful, and I got frequent blood tests. I couldn't go in the sun and was very careful about sleep and self-care. If I didn't sleep, I would suffer migraines.

It was during medical school that things began to fall apart. Doctors generally recommend that people with autoimmune disorders do not go to medical school because of the impact stress and sleep deprivation has on health. But I was determined to fulfill my dream. In the third year of medical school, students have terrible hours, working 100-hour stressful weeks. During my fourth year, I had a severe relapse. I started to get double vision, and I collapsed in the clinic one day. I woke up alone and drove home disoriented and confused. When I woke up again from sleeping at home, I could feel something was very wrong. Tests revealed I had developed anticardiolipin antibodies that were causing blood clots. These blood clots were passing into my brain and causing double vision and a transient ischemic attack, also known as a mini stroke.

My doctors told me I would be at serious risk for a major stroke for the rest of my life, and that I probably wouldn't live to be 50. This is a common diagnosis for people with lupus, which is considered a chronic, progressive disease. My doctors also warned me that since pregnancy is a hyper-coagulable state, that trying to have children would likely result in miscarriages or other fetal injuries and could very likely result in my own death from a major stroke or pulmonary embolism. I was told that I would have to inject myself with blood thinner for the rest of my life.

I spent two weeks mourning the rest of my life. Then I decided to go to a place of gratitude. I was grateful there were medicines that could keep me alive. I decided I would go back and finish medical school. I would be positive, and I wouldn't let anything stop me from finishing my dream.

After graduation, I met a man named Thomas Tadlock. He is the most remarkable human being I have ever met. After only one month, he proposed marriage. I knew with every cell of my being that he was the one I wanted to spend my life with, but I had to make sure he understood what he was getting into, marrying someone with lupus. I told him that I was not going to live a long life, and I couldn't have his children. He would have to take care of me at some point as I became increasingly disabled by the disease. With tears in his eyes, he told me he would rather have a short life with me than a lifetime with anyone else. He was all in.

Again, I was living in a place of celebration and gratitude. How many people get to experience love like this? However short my life would be, I would never want to exchange it with anyone else's. I felt like the luckiest person alive.

At that time, Thomas was a physical trainer and a rapid body transformation specialist working with MTV. I was a medical intern, eating hospital junk food all the time, and ironically the best way to get sick and fat. I was overweight and not in good shape. I desperately wanted to fit into my wedding dress, so I asked him to train me and create a nutrition plan that would make me look as good as his MTV clients.

I had been vegetarian since childhood because of my love for animals, but I wasn't a healthy eater; I was addicted to cheese and ate a lot of processed foods. At that time, he included some meat in his nutrition plans for his clients, for rapid fat loss and fitness transformations. However, because I was a vegetarian, he skipped the meat. He created a nutrition plan for me that had high amounts of raw plant foods, no dairy products because of their high caloric content, no meat, and no processed foods. I went from an unhealthy vegetarian to a high raw food vegan in no time.

What happened next was beyond remarkable. I went from a size 11 to a size 3 in four months. I was super fit and super healthy. And I was able to fit into the wedding dress! More importantly, for the first time in my life, I had no joint pain and no migraines. I was full of energy, despite working 30 straight hours.

I had a blood test before my wedding, only four months after changing my diet. My lupus tests came back negative. My anti-DSDNA antibodies were negative, my complement was normal (which had not happened since my diagnosis

12 years before). My anticardiolipin blood clotting tests were only on the high side of normal. My doctor assumed there had been a mistake at the lab. He asked me to take a blood test again.

When I came back from my honeymoon, the blood tests were repeated. My blood work was still negative for lupus, and my cholesterol and blood pressure had also come down. The anticardiolipin antibodies were negative as well. We were confused. There was no explanation for what had happened, so we called it a remission. It was an unheard-of dramatic remission but being healed was not something we ever considered. I had graduated medical school the year before, so it truly never crossed my mind that diet could impact my disease. After all, I would have learned that in medical school, wouldn't I?

Of course, when lupus goes into remission the blood tests will still reflect the autoimmune condition. Mine didn't. But what else could it all mean? So, I just celebrated my wonderful results and continued doing what I was doing, working long hours for my residency, eating my vegetables, drinking my water, exercising, and spending any spare time with my love. I continued to have monthly appointments with a rheumatologist because I had been doing that for years, but now I was negative for lupus every time. One day he told a medical student accompanying him that I "allegedly" had lupus, but he couldn't find it!

I went on this way for a year before he finally agreed to stop my medications. The idea of taking a lupus patient, who had experienced a mini stroke, off blood thinners gave him enormous anxiety. This, even though I was testing negative for the antibodies. I agreed to come back immediately at any sign of illness. This was in 2006. Since then, I have been completely off all medications, with healthy blood work that has only gotten better over the years.

After this miraculous turn of events, I decided I wanted to have kids. I had been healthy for four years and saw no reason to expect my symptoms to return. My doctors were alarmed and told me that having a baby could bring the lupus back and cause a major stroke, kidney failure or even kill me. My family and friends were frightened, and my best friend offered to carry the baby for me. But I felt strong and healthy, so my husband and I got pregnant.

My obstetrician panicked when I told her "I used to have lupus" during our first meeting. She told me, "That's not possible. You either have lupus, or you don't!" I told her I had it for 12 years but had been negative for 4 years. She sent me to the high-risk obstetrician, but he sent me right back to her, saying he would not take my case because I was perfectly healthy. She watched over me carefully, and I delivered my first child by C-section in 2009. The lupus did not come back. I had another child four years later. Both times I was healthy and had healthy babies. Both times I was effortlessly back in my pre-pregnancy clothes in under two weeks, just sitting around nursing my babies. My body wants to be healthy, strong, and lean.

After the birth of my first child, my husband and I realized that my body was not the same. Not only did the lupus not come back, but my physical recovery was extraordinary as well. We realized that I was not in remission. I was healed.

The only thing that had changed was my diet. We had to figure out what we did so we could replicate it to help others. We are both scientists, and we spent the next year studying cellular biology and how different foods could affect inflammation and immune function. We realized that we had accidentally created an anti-inflammatory diet. We started testing people with chronic diseases on this nutrition plan to see if similar healing takes place.

We were blown away. People have been able to reverse autoimmune diseases such as lupus, scleroderma, rheumatoid arthritis, Sjogren's disease, multiple sclerosis, Reynaud's disease, as well as heart disease, diabetes, and cancer. We realized that this was what we needed to dedicate our lives to: teaching people the power of food, to give them back their life.

In 2012, I retired from my position as the medical director for a wellness center in southern California to focus full time on disease reversal. Now my work is entirely online: I use Skype, phone, Facetime, and other modalities to connect with people from all over the world who need help recovering their health.

After practicing this way for a couple years, I realized that many people need more support, so I created a six-week rapid recovery program where I help people aggressively pursue health through nutrition and lifestyle. I give them daily support and feedback, as much as they need to produce the most rapid results possible. I call it the Health Olympics!

The people graduating these programs have made remarkable recoveries. These include reversing rheumatoid arthritis pain in a few weeks; reversing lupus nephritis by increasing GFR from 14% to 27% in 6 weeks, and thereby preventing the need for a kidney transplant; taking someone from daily seizures of CNS lupus with a DSDNA antibody count of 3300, to being seizure free with a DSDNA count of under 100 in 6 weeks; reversing crippling scleroderma in a young man who went from considering finger amputation to becoming a featured artist in galleries in Los Angeles; and so many more miraculous recoveries. The nutrition plan works rapidly, consistently, and reliably, and every time I am in tears when people recover their health, and more importantly, go on to live lives with meaning, purpose, and joy.

I am committed to spreading the message of health and healing and the power of plants as far and wide as I can. I believe health should be a right, and I will never stop working for everyone to get the health and life they deserve.

Brooke Goldner, M.D.

MY FRESH START WITH FRESH FOODS, AT AGE 27

DOMINIQUE LINDEN

Conditions: Obesity, addiction, alcoholism, depression, brain fog

As a certified yoga teacher and massage therapist, Dominique Linden has been helping people for years. She was a host for PBNSG, the Plant-based Nutrition Support Group, and has shared her plant-based journey on the Forks Over Knives Official Plant-based Group on Facebook. After converting to a whole plant food lifestyle, lifestyle factors such as sobriety, exercise, and sleep have become paramount to Dominique. You can reach her at: **www.bitesizedfaith.com**.

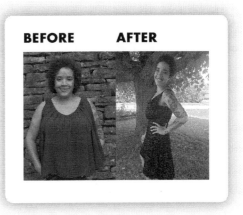

BEFORE   AFTER

I will never forget the night I learned about whole food plant-based eating. I knew vegetarians and vegans existed, but I viewed that lifestyle as a means of protecting animals. I never related it to better health. When I watched the documentary, *Forks Over Knives* that night, I experienced genuine hope and a desire to start living a better life. Here were people getting healthy right before my eyes, and all they had to do was change how they ate. I was all in.

One month before that night I had found myself in a doctor's office. For the first time I openly admitted to a stranger that I was hopelessly depressed and afraid. I finally said those freeing words: "I don't know what to do."

I was only 27, constantly tired, and over 200 pounds. I avoided looking in the mirror whenever possible, and after a lifetime of feeling like I did not belong in my own skin, I was ready for one, last ditch effort to get better before giving up. To feel like you have nothing to look forward to before the age of 30 is very sad and grim. The doctor suggested I eat better, exercise and find a therapist.

The therapy I started right away but eating better and exercising seemed daunting. I had tried and failed so many times before, why would this time be any different? But after learning about a whole food, plant-based (WFPB) lifestyle, I felt deep down that this was it, the answer I had been looking for. The science made sense to me, the studies fascinated me, and the simple concept of eating more whole foods to feel better helped me make sense of why I had always felt the way I had. The cherry on top of this WFPB sundae was when I told my new therapist about the *Forks Over Knives* documentary I had watched. She happily exclaimed that she ate that way, too. A whole food, plant-based diet had reversed her diabetes. We still share recipes.

As obvious as it seems now, the fact that what I ate affected the quality of my life was foreign to me. I had eaten whatever I wanted, whenever I wanted. And what I mostly wanted was red meat, tons of cheese and a daily sugar binge (or two or three). I would eat late at night. Some days I would starve myself most of the day so I could overeat later. I ate packaged food or fast food for almost every single meal. I ate when I was bored, sad, happy, nervous, or in pain. Nutrition and wellbeing were not things we discussed growing up, so this was all normal to me.

The magical timing of hitting rock bottom and watching *Forks Over Knives* was just what I needed to realize that to change a lifetime of bad habits, I was going to need to start somewhere. I stopped eating out, and only cooked at home. I bought multiple WFPB cookbooks and joined online support groups. As I started to lose weight and feel better, two things in my life became painfully apparent; not only had I eaten whatever I wanted, I also drank and smoked whatever I wanted. Once again, it seems obvious now that those things would affect my life, but I had not been able to face the truth until I started to feel better about myself.

The constant brain fog I had experienced since I was little started to lift. I felt energetic and light for the first time ever. And because of this newfound hope, it became easier to look at the rest of my life and see that, really, none of it was working out too well. Five months into my plant-based life, I quit smoking cigarettes after years of trying to stop. A month after that, I had my last alcoholic drink when realizing that alcohol was a problem in my life.

Three months later, I left the longest relationship that I had ever been in, knowing it was not good for either of us. All those changes were extremely hard but experiencing the benefits of a whole food, plant-based lifestyle kept me going. I also continued my therapy and slowly learned to face my fears and depression, instead of running from them like I always had.

Today, almost 3 years later, I have lost almost 40 pounds, and my BMI has gone from 32 to 26. Even though harder moments have happened in my life than ever before, depression does not feel like it has the power to take me out anymore. I can honestly say that I have never felt this comfortable in my own skin, or this content. My weight still fluctuates, I still give in to emotional eating sometimes. But today, I have a baseline of hope instead of a baseline of feeling defeated. I know eating this way works.

I eat like I love myself, and because of that I am learning to love myself. I was able to see more clearly what alcohol and drugs do to me because of the clarity I gained from eating better, and today I know I want nothing to do with them. Depression, addiction, and childhood trauma are all part of my story, and they are why I have needed this trio of plant-based eating, sobriety, and therapy to get better.

But today I know that is not where my story ends. Today I know there is always a chance to turn your life around.

My fresh start started with fresh foods.

Dominique Linden

FROM DISTRESSED GUT TO HARMONIZED HAPPINESS

MELISSA MONDALA M.D.

Conditions: Irritable Bowel Syndrome, GERD, acne, anxiety, overweight, depression

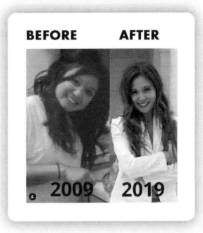

Dr. Melissa Mondala obtained her medical degree from Chicago Medical School. She has 3 medical specialties – family medicine, primary care psychiatry and lifestyle medicine. She served as an Associate Professor of Medicine at Loma Linda University and developed a lifestyle medical clinic in San Bernardino, CA. Dr. Mondala has been featured in several publications and has spoken about the science of plant-based nutrition and mental health at different venues. She and her husband, Dr. Micha Yu, co-founded a lifestyle and integrative clinic in Newport Beach, CA called "Dr. Lifestyle."
See Dr. Micah Yu's story elsewhere in this book. Dr. Mondala is highly passionate about the science of nutrition and sees patients in person or via telemedicine at: **www.drlifestyle.org**.

Behind a successful career was my disordered, stressed gut.

As a young girl, I watched my dad struggle with the autoimmune skin disease, psoriasis. Steroids and other medications were not providing relief or resolving it. As with most diseases, underlying root causes were not being addressed. Finally, my dad discovered the Dr. McDougall diet for his health and the solutions he needed to heal.

Still in my teens, I could not imagine nor wanted to believe that my dad's new diet could possibly be a lifestyle for me, even though I was also living with chronic disease. I suffered from severe stomach cramps, acne, and emotional stress. I did not accept that I was truly sick like my father. It was not until years later, as an adult, that I would finally address my own health issues.

Over the years, I had crawled on the floor because of those severe stomach cramps and a pregnant-sized belly full of gas. I would often run to the toilet, sometimes barely making it in time. I was too ashamed to tell anyone of these recurrences. I thought it was normal because I believed, "I simply ate too fast."

I coped by eating Tums and Pepcid like candy, just so I could continue to get by eating my favorite foods. Those foods were often hot Cheetos, white chocolate, and ice cream. I was a thin cheerleader captain who was very active and loved eating competitions with the football and basketball players. I would yell, dance, and lead my team into "school spirit." I saw myself as strong and able to digest large amounts of food no matter how fatty, spicy, or salty.

I often gulped down a standard Filipino diet with roasted pork, fried chicken, beef steak, and heavy seafood. After meals, I developed a burning in my belly that would rise into my chest. At the time, I thought it was a sign of being satisfied and having a good meal or what others would call the "meat sweats." Little did I know that the food would inflame my body. I also struggled with acne during the same time, going through rounds of topical and oral medication with no improvement.

As time progressed, I combined the standard American diet (SAD) with the standard Filipino diet. I was in medical school, eating meat lover pizzas, BBQ meats, and hot dogs; and gaining weight, I loved food and food loved me. Or so I thought. Soon however, I became sensitive to dairy, then to other foods and finally, even to cold water and ice. I kept pushing through all these symptoms because I was focused on getting through medical school, having no time to stop and look at my own health.

On the surface, many saw me as thriving. I was juggling multiple student organizations, various presidential and leadership roles, two part-time jobs and the maximum number of school credits with a breeze. Yet, I was living with uncontrollable symptoms of GERD, acne, anxiety, and irritable bowel syndrome (IBS). I noticed that my mood, focus, performance, and gut suffered tremendously. I became extremely sensitive to all foods. I would get frequent diarrhea, bloating, abdominal cramps. I was highly inflamed. I soon missed out on social activities and was very unhappy. My acne and irritable bowel syndrome worsened.

As a medical student at Loma Linda University, where I did my residency, I met Dr. Brenda Rea, who told me her own story of healing her multiple sclerosis. She explained to me that lifestyle is the first line of defense and the way to reverse ill health. I began reading scientific articles and the book, *How Not to Die* by Dr. Michael Gregor. I watched the documentary films, *Forks Over Knives,* and *What the Health?* I attended many plant-based conferences including the *International Plant based Nutrition Health Conference*. I was hooked on the strong scientific evidence and the health transformation possibilities.

Initially, I decided to start my lifestyle change by running. I began to "run off" the symptoms, exercising regularly, and training for 5k and 10k runs. With exercise, and cutting out processed foods and reducing my stress, my IBS improved about 50 percent. However, that still was only 50 percent. I finally decided to go all in — totally whole food, plant-based.

I lost 15 pounds, which for a small framed woman, is a game changer! And I gained the best long-lasting benefits; my acne, GERD, and IBS resolved for the first time ever. I was transformed!

I soon had amazing energy throughout the day, a new laser focus, and a resilient, upbeat mood! I no longer had anxiety or depression to pull me down.

I followed Dr. Scott Stoll, the co-author of this book, and his team at the Plantrician Project. I appreciate his amplifying the evidence of whole food plant-based science in health. It has been a complete mind and heart shift for me. I didn't want to suffer with IBS all my life as a physician. I learned that there is a better solution than a temporary band aid fix with medications. I am a completely different person, as is my husband, Dr. Micah Yu, who has his own story of healing in this book.

We embraced the plant-based lifestyle together. We read labels, look for the salt, sugar, and fiber content in everything we eat. After multiple pantry and fridge dumps, we replaced our old unhealthy food with fresh fruits, vegetables, beans, lentils, and whole grains. We found new spices, herbs, and condiments. Today we use simple plant-based recipe books and find recipes. We also enjoy how others also cook plant-based foods. Every day, I am thankful for this lifestyle and my body.

I had come to recognize the negative self-talk and self-destructive behaviors that I had been living with for so long. Those are now gone. There is no turning back. The results are real and lasting!

Today, I enjoy helping my peers and patients deal with their life crises including family issues, divorce, academic failure, and depression. I have learned that statistically, 50 percent of most patients with depression are often misdiagnosed by their doctors. And once they are diagnosed, they do not necessarily respond to the medication as a stand-alone treatment. This led me to pursue the gut brain connection in mental health.

Today, using a whole food-based diet and cardiovascular exercise, my patients with depression are improving a minimum of 50 percent. Additionally, I encourage sleep hygiene, stress management and a focus on gratitude and resilience.

As expected, many of my patients also have other addictions: food, drugs, alcohol, smoking, and shopping. This new, plant-based lifestyle allows them to pursue a complete holistic care program in every area of their lives, giving them a new sense of purpose and control.

Plants are the go-to for everything. Plants are my healing tools for patients. My patients are now experiencing an enjoyable, purposeful lifestyle, adding days to their lives living better for their loved ones, children, parents, siblings, friends, and neighbors. I empower my patients every day telling them all to "be consistent, be mindful, and be patient. Your future self will thank you!"

My mantra is:
"One cannot think well, love well, sleep well, if one has not dined well."
Virginia Woolf, "A Room of One's Own."

Melissa Mondala, M.D.

FROM RHEUMATOLOGY PATIENT TO RHEUMATOLOGY HEALER

MICAH YU, M.D.

Conditions: Rheumatoid arthritis, spondyloarthritis, gout, overweight

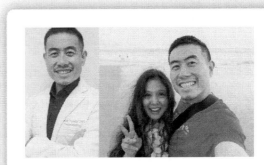

Dr. Micah Yu. Dr. Melissa Mondala & Dr. Micah Yu

Dr. Micah Yu is board-certified in both internal medicine and lifestyle medicine. He specializes in integrative rheumatology treatment incorporating plant-based nutrition, as well as traditional rheumatology approaches. He obtained his medical degree from the Chicago Medical School and is an Assistant Professor of Medicine at the California University of Science and Medicine. He speaks frequently at conferences and at the American College of Rheumatology. Dr. Yu's focus on rheumatological diseases stems from his own ordeals with arthritis, gout and spondyloarthritis (arthritis of the spine and large joints). He is in private practice at the clinic he co-founded with his wife, Dr. Melissa Mondala, in Newport Beach, CA called "Dr. Lifestyle." See Dr. Melissa Mondala's story elsewhere in this book. Dr. Yu sees patients in person or via telemedicine at **www.drlifestyle.org**.

You don't expect to have arthritis as a teenager, but that's exactly what I have battled since the age of 17.

Growing up I ate a very typical standard American diet (SAD). Chips, chicken nuggets, soda, double cheeseburgers, hot dogs, etc. I also ate unhealthy Asian food that included lots of fried and oily food. I was overweight and getting heavier and unhealthier every year.

I was a football player in my high school. At 5'5" and 160 pounds, I was playing as a defensive lineman in my sophomore year of high school. Being slow and overweight, that was the only position I could play. After a year of high school football, I got stronger and developed a passion for lifting weights.

However, I wanted to also lose weight at the same time, since I was fed up with being overweight. I searched and searched and came upon the Atkins diet. This was a diet that was very popular in the decades of 1990 and 2000. After doing a lot of research, I made it a mission to get as much protein into my body as possible, eating as much as 160-200 grams of protein per day. I ate steak, fish, protein shakes, dairy, chicken, and ham to get the protein in. I ate very little carbohydrates. In a matter of months, I was able to lose 20 to 30 pounds and gain more muscle mass and strength as well. I was very proud of my accomplishment. The Atkins diet was doing its job.

In the fall of 2003, I woke up one night with excruciating pain on my right big toe. It felt like someone used a piece of wood to slam my toe in the middle of the night. My toe was red, hot, swollen and throbbing. I could not walk and was on the verge of crying. I ended up limping to school the same day. My father, who is a family physician, got lab tests done on me and eventually diagnosed it as gout. My uric acid was 13 at the time of diagnosis (normal is 3.4 - 7.0). I was given a dietary plan for gout that limited my protein intake.

I stopped the Atkins diet quickly after the diagnosis but that did not stop me from continuing to eat the SAD diet. During college, I had repeated gout flares and it made socializing very difficult as I would have to avoid social functions. My gout would seem to flare from every couple of months to almost every month. I then started medication for my gout, which seemed to help.

However, prior to starting medical school, I developed arthritis, which spread to more and more joints with more and more pain. I started getting pain in the TMJs of my jaws, as well as my wrists, hands, knees, ankles, and feet. There was a time when I had to skip school for two weeks straight while I was bedridden from all the pain. During medical school, I went to several rheumatologists. They did not know what other disease was manifesting besides my gout. My autoimmune antibodies were all negative, but my inflammatory markers were persistently elevated.

I remember when my TMJs would be so swollen that I could not eat anything other than yogurt and fluids, for weeks on end. The only minor relief I could get was by taking pain medication and going to sleep. People would see me limping to school. I was a 24-year-old man stuck in an 80-year-old body. Staying out late to hang out with my friends sometimes meant a week of pain. Morning stiffness was common.

One of the worst places for flares and attacks would be my feet, especially the bottom of my feet. Sometimes it would feel like the bottom of my feet were on fire. The bones would throb. I would put a lot of pressure on my foot and press it hard into the ground, just to get some relief from the pain. How could someone so young be suffering from so much pain and swelling? It didn't make sense!

As I transitioned to internal medicine residency at Loma Linda University, I started seeking out the medical care of the rheumatologists there. I was hopeful that someone would be able to find some answers. One day my knee started flaring and I headed over to the rheumatology clinic. A quick ultrasound of my knee revealed that I had inflammation of my tendons. I was told that I had something called enthesitis, which is inflammation of the entheses (the connection point between the bone and tendons).

My diagnosis was spondyloarthritis, a type of autoimmune arthritis. I was offered to start medications such as hydroxychloroquine and methotrexate, but I refused. I did not want to be on medications even though I was already on gout medication. Being in your 20s and having to face the possibility of taking medication for possibly your entire life was not attractive to me.

I noticed that my pain would wax and wane with certain foods, but I could not pinpoint it. I was hopeful that one day I would be able to figure it out and not need medications.

One of the worst memories of pain that would never escape me was when I was on my ICU rotation as an intern and had an attack on my left hip. I literally had to grab my left leg to lift it into the car to get to work. From there, I would limp all the way to the ICU. Making the rounds of the ICU would take hours. The attending physician doing the ICU rounds with me had to give me a chair to sit in because I looked so uncomfortable. This went on for two weeks straight. I was scared that I wouldn't be able to finish residency because of my pain. I hated it and didn't know if I would need a cane or crutches going into a few years when I would be in my 30s.

Fortunately, my wife, Dr. Melissa Mondala, whose story is elsewhere in this book, started exploring Lifestyle Medicine at Loma Linda University during our residency. It was during the 3rd and last year of our residency that she got introduced to a plant-based lifestyle. She made some plant-based dishes during Thanksgiving. I did not like the food at all.

Several months went by, and I ended up buying the book, *How Not to Die*, by Dr. Michael Greger. We both went to Guam for our medical rotation for a month. At the Guam clinic, all the food was vegetarian. I started getting used to the food, and How Not to Die was quite inspirational. I came back to California and watched the documentary film, *Forks Over Knives*. It was then that I decided to change my diet and go plant-based to see if this diet would change the outcome of my disease. Within 3 months of converting to a whole food, plant-based diet, I lost 10 pounds and my pain went away completely. I was shocked.

Blood work showed that my C-reactive protein (a marker of inflammation) went completely negative after being positive for almost 10 years. I didn't even know if I had the disease anymore. I had no flares in three months. This was a miracle for me!

No one ever discussed diet and nutrition with me at all. Not one doctor ever did that! Nor was it discussed in medical school. Nor in my residency. How could something as simple as proper nutrition fix my problems? I couldn't believe it.

Because of my own pain and disease, I decided to specialize in rheumatology very early in my medical career. Not only did I want to understand my own diseases, but I also wanted to help patients who suffered like I did.

As I went through my fellowship, I shared the good news of proper nutrition and a whole food, plant-based diet with my patients and colleagues. I saw patients get better and some even get off medications. I shared my own personal experience with them, that it is possible to get better with just a healthier diet. With this new discovery, I opened a clinic with my wife called "Dr. Lifestyle" in Newport Beach, California. We use lifestyle medicine as the foundation of our clinic.

I recently obtained my lab results. My ESR (another inflammatory marker) went completely negative after 10 years of being positive. If I eat the wrong foods, such as highly processed foods when eating out, then I can potentially get some pain. However, 99% of the time I don't get any pain, and when the pain does come it is only 10% of the pain or less of the pain that I used to experience, and it goes away within a day.

I don't take medications for my spondyloarthritis, but I still take medication for gout. Spondyloarthritis is an autoimmune disease whereas gout is not. However, it is possible that the gout flares can eventually go away if one stays fastidiously on a whole food, plant-based diet.[1]

Today, I use my personal experience, along with my never-ending thirst for knowledge of integrative/lifestyle medicine and autoimmune diseases, to help my patients in our clinic and share the good word through social media. A plant-based diet can potentially put autoimmune disease into reversal.

I am so happy that I have experienced this personally as a physician.

Micah Yu, M.D.

[1] The authors of this book, Dan Purjes and Scott Stoll, M.D., are aware of cases where gout was completely reversed through a whole plant food diet that was adhered to for a long enough period of time.

MY FATHER'S CANCER LED ME TO BE A PLANT-BASED DOCTOR

RON WEISS, M.D.

Condition: Pancreatic cancer, obesity, diabetes (all pertaining to Dr. Weiss' father)

Ron Weiss, M.D., is a physician and a regenerative farmer. He is dual board-certified in internal medicine and lifestyle medicine. Dr. Weiss is Assistant Professor of Clinical Medicine at Rutgers Medical School in New Jersey. His practice, Ethos Primary Care, is located at Ethos Farm, a 300-year-old working farm in Long Valley, NJ.

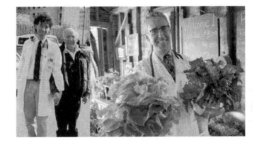

Dr. Ron Weiss & father   Dr. Ron Weiss at Ethos Farm

To obtain plant-based care visit: **www.EthosPrimaryCare.com**.

Dr Weiss is also the founder of the Ethos Farm Project, a farm-based, non-profit healthcare system. The Ethos Farm Project took two broken American systems – food and healthcare – and merged them. The new system seeks to restore the health of the community and protect the health of the earth. Ethos Farm Project's objectives are to feed the community, train regenerative farmers and lifestyle medicine physicians, educate the public and promote climate change solutions through the restoration of agricultural soils. Ethos Farm is certified organic and employs chemical-free regenerative farming methods to restore the vitality of the land.

To find out more, visit **www.EthosFarmProject.org**.

My father was born of deprivation. His arrival into the world in Poland, 1922, followed the death of two brothers. His mother told him they died as toddlers during World War I of malnutrition.

My father himself had little to eat, growing up in what was to become the Lódz Ghetto of Poland. One of the delights of his childhood was when his mother, my grandmother, would take him to the forest at the edge of the city to buy him a "stonik." Stoniks were little pastries filled with the wild blueberries that grew in the woods. The little cakes were dusted with confectioner's sugars and sold by vendors from carts in the forest. Grandmother would save up all year long to buy him a stonik.

By the time he emigrated to America with my grandmother on the eve of the Holocaust, my father was 14 years old and weighed less than 100 lbs. They came to Paterson, NJ, where my grandfather had settled a few years earlier. My grandfather sold women's underwear door to door during the Great Depression and scraped up enough money to buy them tickets for the steamship passage.

At age 14, my dad entered kindergarten in the Paterson public schools because he spoke no English. But 4 years later, he graduated from Eastside High school with honors. He was drafted into the Army Air Corps and was sent back to Europe to fight in the Battle of the Bulge.

After the war, my dad attended Rutgers University, and then Rutgers Law School. He was the first person in his family ever to get a higher education. He opened his law practice in Paterson, married my mother and raised a family of six children, three of whom became physicians.

Having full access to the bounty of post war America, Dad started to gain weight in his 30s and 40s. He ate an omnivorous diet with a focus on seafood as well as traditional Italian and Jewish delicacies. My father derived intense joy from eating delicious food, perhaps stemming from his meager origins. Among the favorite foods he would eat regularly were escarole and beans with large amounts of garlic, ossobuco and other veal dishes, broiled fish of all sorts, calamari, clams, oysters, smoked whitefish. He loved traditional Jewish foods such as herring and bagels, lox, and cream cheese. By the time he reached his 50s, my father was obese, weighing 210 lbs, and he was diagnosed with diabetes.

He had also taken up the habit of smoking a cigar a day. He was physically active for most of his life, enjoying gym workouts, swimming, tennis and walking daily. He began to slim down a bit in his late 60s, losing about 30 lbs, but it was not clear that this was intentional.

About the time of his 70th birthday he began to experience severe constant abdominal pains. This was very unusual for him. Abdominal cat scans revealed a large mass on the pancreas, with extensive liver metastases. A biopsy revealed pancreatic adenocarcinoma - cancer of the pancreas.

I had recently finished my medical training and was a practicing physician in California. I decided to move back home to take care of my father. With an impending sense of doom, my physician brothers and I took our father for a second opinion to New York's best cancer hospital.

The doctor gave us a grim prognosis: Dad had a few months left. We were offered the standard chemotherapy at the time which was 5-fluorouracil. It afforded no discernible survival benefit yet caused significant side effects, so my father refused it. The doctor gave him a Percocet prescription for pain control and advised him to go home and get his affairs in order.

As we left the hospital, it felt as if the world were ending. Knowing how much our father loved Jewish deli, we took him to a lunch of comfort food at the Carnegie Deli. In the past we had visited Carnegie Deli as a special treat on joyous occasions. Now we sat before the beloved pastrami and corned beef sandwiches piled up high and swallowed them in silence. A dirge played in our heads. Little did I understand that we were feeding my father the very food that caused his cancer.

I can only describe the next week at home with my dad as "the unbearable heaviness of being." Even though I was a newly minted doctor with the most up-to-date information and skills, I felt completely powerless to help my own father. I had taken care of many patients with stage 4 pancreatic cancer in my residency. All of them died a miserable, painful death within a year or less. Seeking to learn anything other than what I already knew about end-stage cancer patients, I left the house one day and went down to the public library in town. It was the early 90s and alternative medicine was becoming all the rage.

I spent days in the library reading all kinds of books on alternative therapies I knew nothing about Chinese herbs, acupuncture, Ayurvedic medicine, etc. But then I saw a book about using food as medicine, and food was something familiar to me. The book contained testimonies of people with dire illnesses who had reversed them by eating a macrobiotic diet, which is a type of diet of whole plant foods. In this book, I read about Norman Arnold, who had successfully overcome stage 4 pancreatic cancer using a macrobiotic diet. This inspired Mr. Arnold to create an endowment at the University of South Carolina School of Public Health, which is today named after him.

I read Mr. Arnold's story to my father and he was interested. So, I took him to see a dietician in West Orange, NJ by the name of Elaine Nussbaum who had adopted a macrobiotic diet a decade earlier to treat her own uterine carcinosarcoma. The disease was usually metastatic to the lungs and spine, yet it resolved completely.

Next, I took my father to Boston to be evaluated by Elaine's mentor and leader of the macrobiotic movement, Michio Kushi. Mr. Kushi placed my father on the most severely restricted diet we could ever imagine, consisting primarily of dark leafy cruciferous greens, a variety of other vegetables, legumes, brown rice and other selected grains like buckwheat and millet, mushrooms, and seaweed. Strictly forbidden were all plants of the nightshade family; potatoes, tomatoes, peppers and eggplant, fruit, and foods of animal origin. We also were directed to get rid of all plastic and old cookware and to use only stainless steel. It all seemed quite crazy to me, but it was our only option.

We went from Mr. Kushi's office directly to the Bread and Circus organic market to stock up. As we walked through the parking lot. I remember seeing the gleam of hope in my father's eyes. He smiled for the first time in many weeks, turned to me and said he was going to beat this cancer, and he would dedicate himself fully to the diet.

We started. My mother was the dedicated foot soldier who acquired and prepared all the food. Within 24 hours of starting the diet the constipation my father had been experiencing since his diagnosis, suddenly disappeared. Within a week, he no longer needed the Percocet. His severe abdominal pain was gone. He returned to his law practice. Two weeks later he was back in the gym, three weeks later he was running. He felt so good, so vital and so full of energy.

For the life of me, I just could not understand what was going on - was it the placebo effect? But to see Dad transform before our eyes was exhilarating and filled us all with hope.

Since his diagnosis, his CA 19-9, a pancreatic tumor marker, as well as his liver function tests had been rising quickly and large areas of his liver had already been replaced by tumor. A month after starting the diet, we checked his CA 19-9 and liver function tests, both dropped dramatically!

Three months later, a repeat abdominal CAT scan revealed his major tumor masses had been reduced in size by a third. By this time, his long-standing diabetes had also resolved. At six months, we obtained another CAT scan, which demonstrated a 50% reduction in his major tumor masses!

One year later, my father was still doing well. We took him back to the cancer hospital to check in with the doctor who initially saw him, to find out if any new treatment protocols for pancreatic cancer had become available. When the doctor laid eyes on my father, he seemed startled to see my dad still alive.

We recounted my father's story to the doctor. When we told him the kale, brown rice, seaweed, etc. were responsible for his improvement, the doctor fell silent, as if a wall had suddenly descended between us. Without inquiring further, the doctor abruptly changed the topic of discussion to chemotherapy.

I was dumbfounded. I knew in my physician's heart that it was my father's dietary change that was responsible for shrinking his tumors. This was no magical thinking. Yet this cancer specialist didn't want to hear anything about it. As a young physician, I learned an important lesson that day. Patients are the physician's greatest teachers. The clinician as an acute observer is able to learn from a patient and make new discoveries. All that is required is that he or she listens compassionately and have an open mind and willingness to learn. New revelations can benefit other patients and society through the work of the physician.

I walked out of the doctor visit that day, forever changed as a physician. That was the moment. My life would never be the same again.

After 18 months, my father eventually succumbed to his disease. But for most of that time, he led a high-quality life with his family. I attribute this to his diet of whole plant foods and the hope it provided when there was nothing else but darkness and death. He continued doing what he loved most, practicing law in his little office in a poverty-stricken neighborhood of Paterson, NJ until 2 weeks before his death.

Soon after, I moved out of the house into my own apartment. As I was unpacking boxes, I pulled out my New Jersey Medical School diploma. I lifted it out of the box and held it in the sunlight. I gazed at the diploma's gilded, embossed seal depicting Hippocrates and his staff of Asclepius. In that moment, I realized I knew almost nothing of this man and his teachings, even though I had taken the Hippocratic Oath upon graduation. I went back to the library and learned about Hippocrates' greatest teaching: Food is the most powerful agent of healing.

"Let food be thy medicine," said Hippocrates.

Ever since, I have used food as the primary treatment tool for my patients.

I am often asked this one question. Why did the cancer come back?

I have many insights that I have learned from that, which have brought me along my path as a physician. The key message of this story is that my father was triumphant for the period of time he lived beyond what had been predicted by the oncologist, and that it was quality living, without suffering.

The most powerful aspect of his story and this collection of stories from my perspective as a physician, is that it is humanized, with humbling lessons that it teaches the readers. Life is not always about winning first place. Most of us do not win first place or become champions. As a physician, who is a lifestyle doctor, who treats over 150 patients a week in a very busy clinic, who seeks to heal, and, as a regenerative farmer who is growing organic fruits and vegetables, we take what we are given.

Medicines and other forces are humbling mistresses. This story imparts the feeling that there is vast opportunity and hope, but it is not always realized. There is still grief, there is still pain. People still die. The lesson from this book and many of us who have stories is that one should apply these lessons and travel this road.

There are other treasures that will be realized. With my father, he had extra time. His survival was improved. Conservatively, it quadrupled his survival. No chemo, no treatment could have given him this. He got to be with his family, travelling, going to the gym and was able to practice law in his own office. He was not in pain and was full of energy. He was living better than before cancer. I see this as an enormous benefit.

Even though the cancer came back, and as with many of my other patients, there is victory.

Always, when you want to be effective as a healthcare provider, you must be honest. We *have* to be honest. I have many patients. I tell them my father's story and they know he died. Very few late-stage cancers will be cured but it is possible and that gives great hope.[1] That is what I learned. There is no hope otherwise. It is the idea that there is something that one can do. The overwhelming grief was that there was nothing that could be done ... until there was something, called whole plant food.

Something as simple as food.

My father's story is the connection to what led to the decision to acquire the farm and what we do today at Ethos farm. In many ways, it is beyond our capacity to do what we do.

I looked at so many fields covered in GMO corn and soybean, being fed to animals that were grown to kill people, I imagined my dad standing there in this vast corn field, in the corn rows. I thought, we must change this just as he changed what he did. His image inspired me to change, to reverse cancer and disease, heal people instead of killing them, healing them with food.

That was the deciding moment for me. We had to figure out a way to transition this land that had been poisoned with so many chemicals to grow beautiful food with nature's phytochemicals that fight cancer and other diseases.

Let food be thy medicine!

Ron Weiss, M.D.

---

[1] There are two stories in this book of different late stage, terminal cancers that improved through conversion to a whole plant food diet. In both cases the patients were told they only had a few months left to live.

ASTHMA AWAY!

JACKIE OLMSTEAD

Conditions: Asthma, Irritable Bowel Syndrome (IBS), Hashimoto's disease, celiac disease, hypoglycemia, anemia, vertigo, hormonal imbalances, menstrual problems, fertility problems, panic attacks, overweight, depression

You would think that Jackie Olmstead would have grown up with little to no health issues since her father was a physician and her mother was a nurse. But at six months old, she was diagnosed with asthma. Being hospitalized several times while enduring breathing treatments, steroids, antibiotics, inhalers, and oral asthma medicines was challenging, and a lonely and scary way to grow up. All these treatments, medicines and emergency room visits continued into her forties. Viruses, flu bugs and sometimes exercise would trigger an asthma episode that would last for one to two weeks and occurred twice a year or more. Other diagnoses would emerge later including irritable bowel syndrome (IBS), Hashimoto's disease, hypoglycemia, and depression. She then discovered a whole food, plant-based lifestyle and today no longer owns any inhalers. She has had only one asthma attack in 6 years. Follow Jackie on her blog: **https://earthmommaliving.com**.

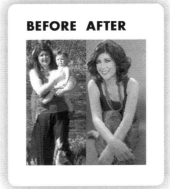

BEFORE   AFTER

As I have grown, I can see now how offering my story and experiences with my health journey can help others. **I never expected to heal my asthma and other health issues by simply changing the way I ate.**

When I lived in Denver as a child, I remember staying up late at night playing in the living room with my younger brother. I was not feeling well, having yet another asthma episode. This was not the first nor the last asthma episode. Taking asthma medicine had several side effects, including speeding up my heart rate, feeling manic and keeping me all too wide awake to go to sleep. Between the medicine and the sickness, I would experience vertigo as well. I had to stay in bed all too often for a young girl and I was so very tired of it.

There were fun times, too, but not without consequence for my natural, playful self. As much as I loved to be outside with my family and friends, I would soon find myself wheezing. I loved the outdoors, playing with my brother on the backyard swing set and with other kids in the neighborhood. We flew kites and went camping with our parents in Colorado's natural and beautiful outdoors. Yet, I always had to be careful as to how much I could play, as typical childhood play would be too strenuous of an activity for my lungs. Even the cold, crisp Colorado air would trigger dreaded wheezing and oftentimes a worse reaction, ending with me back in the hospital again, all just playing!

I remember having pneumonia several times and being confined to an oxygen tent at home. I'll never forget the plastic smell that reminded me of what was helping me breathe better. The nebulizer treatments, antibiotics and asthma pills all worked together to eventually get me on my feet again.

Longer hospital stays started when I was in elementary school. Missing class meant homework sent home from my teachers. I was to do my school assignments on my own at home. It was extremely lonely and overwhelming to do my work in bed, whether at home or in the hospital. I wanted to do well in school, however, and I was determined to get good grades. Thus, I excelled in every subject.

We moved to North Carolina when I was nine. There I began doing gymnastics, always with my inhaler never far away. I loved how it felt to be in great physical shape, finally in control of my body! I could express myself, be creative and excel at a sport that was all my own.

Asthma always returned though, with predictable episodes whenever I got a cold or flu bug. I remember asking my parents, "Can't I please just get a lung transplant?" with tears in my eyes. At 9 or 10, I was so frustrated with all of it: the pain, and the fears of feeling like I might die, I would plead with my dad to help me. He would reply, "No, pumpkin, you can't," and hug me.

As a doctor, my father knew there was little that could be done to help his own daughter. I can only imagine what fears my mom and dad had every time I got sick. They would get up several times at night to check on me, visit me in the hospitals, and do as much as they could. As a parent today, I have a tremendous amount of compassion for them.

Into my teens, nothing got better with my asthma. In fact, things got worse for my health. I was diagnosed with irritable bowel syndrome (IBS). Today, I believe what contributed to my diseased digestive system were all the medications I took my entire life. Certainly, that coupled with the unhealthy foods I ate then played a large part in how miserable I felt.

By high school, we had moved multiple times, and we were now living in Pennsylvania. Depression added to my health struggles, including a deepening sense of loneliness. This led to therapists who could offer some emotional support but no real solutions for my chronic health crises and now my mental health was at risk.

I continued exercising with aerobics after having quit competitive gymnastics when I was twelve. My grades were beginning to suffer somewhat compared to my earlier years as my health issues were piling up. However, I still successfully got into Pennsylvania State University.

When I got to Penn State, I immediately began drinking excessively. I even tried smoking. UGH! I don't like to think of these days in my life. They were dark.

I often thought to myself I didn't want to be here on this earth anymore. I had gained a bunch of weight very fast, no doubt due to the drinking and the standard college diet. I was puffy, swollen, and miserable. Still driven, and a perfectionist, I leaned on my schooling to power me through those days so that I could feel like I mattered. But, my reality was showing up hungover in class, often late, hiding in the back row, and falling asleep. This was humiliating for me, as I was a conscientious student. I had no idea how my health was impacting my choices and my choices impacting my health.

I had started out in an engineering program as I had excelled in the sciences and math, yet I soon discovered I genuinely preferred graphic design and the arts. After finishing those four years of education, I decided to do something completely different, adding a study-abroad experience to my curriculum. For an additional two semesters, I studied art, Italian literature, and the Italian language in central Italy.

To manage my asthma, I packed plenty of steroids and inhalers to take with me to Europe. I loved Italy. This was one of the best educational and personal decisions I made in my own life. Seeing how the Italians cherish their families, how they prepared food slowly, devoting their energy to their meals along with learning about other cultures was priceless. I learned more about what I wanted, which included joy and a sense of wellbeing. I knew it was up to me.

Still struggling with breathing, I finally had to go to a clinic and discovered they did not have the same asthma medicines that were in the United States. I survived. Barely well enough to return home to graduate, still chronically ill with asthma, IBS and depression, I needed a change. But I did not know what it was going to be.

Armed with a degree in graphic design, I got my first official job in New York City in 1990. This was a milestone year. You would think that I would be over-the-moon and proud of myself, having "made it" with such an excellent graphics job at one of the major national magazines in New York City. I also had my own apartment. But I was not elated. All the drinking and my lifestyle in college to cope with my health and depression came to a grinding halt! I was very distressed.

I stayed in New York for five years. It got to the point where I was so ill and so depressed not knowing how to feel better, I felt like I didn't want to live any more, or at least not like this any longer. Restless in New York, I now knew I had to make a life change. Wanting a healthier life and place to live, I moved to Phoenix, Arizona in 1995. I have lived there ever since. There, I would experience the most important shifts, growths, and losses in my life.

In 1999, while in Arizona, I met my future husband. We married in 2006. I soon had significant trouble getting and staying pregnant despite very much wanting to become a mother. The doctors discovered my hormones were not balanced nor did they believe my hormone levels were conducive to having a full-term pregnancy or a healthy baby. At first, I was told I had too much prolactin, in part due to my pituitary gland showing a benign tumor on an MRI. Medication and time would eventually balance the hormone, and the tumor subsided so as not to be a factor. But the excess prolactin was also the cause of ongoing menstrual irregularity, impacting my fertility.

Then, finally, in 2007, after suffering four painful and heartbreaking miscarriages over the course of two years, the doctors finally discovered I also had Hashimoto's disease. They prescribed Synthroid to treat it. Soon thereafter, my doctors also diagnosed hypoglycemia. I started to follow a more intentional diet to manage the hypoglycemia, with small meals every two hours. But I did not yet know the best foods for my body.

In 2008, to everyone's delight, especially mine, I finally gave birth to a perfectly healthy, beautiful, baby girl. I had spent the years addressing my hormone struggles researching how to have the healthiest pregnancy and birth experience. Still, my life was not settled, and my marriage was in trouble.

My mother passed away in 2011 and things were still not going well with my marriage. I was clinically depressed and started taking antidepressants. Unfortunately, my marriage did not work out and we divorced in 2013. I was still dealing with my health, now on my own as a single mother with a young child.

Depression persisted as did the grief of my mother's death and the end of my marriage. One of my nurse friends soon noticed that I was now eating cups of ice one after another daily. She told me, "That is a symptom of anemia. You should get that checked out immediately, Jackie!" I did and learned I also had anemia.

My father had always helped me learn how to do my own patient advocacy by asking my own doctors many questions. I would ask for appropriate tests, finding new doctors if the ones I was seeing didn't listen to me or refused to keep searching for what was really going on with me medically. With the right doctors, I got comprehensive blood work plus a small intestine biopsy that confirmed I had celiac disease and severe anemia.

The hematologist ordered urgent intravenous iron transfusions and prescription strength vitamin D and folic acid. Once a week for five weeks, I would sit for an hour in the same room cancer patients received their chemotherapy treatments. It was bizarre because I didn't feel like I belonged there but knew it would help me heal.

I was so relieved to finally know what was wrong with me, but then, I was in shock and anxious about what to do now with celiac disease. How on earth do I cut out 100% of all the gluten from my life overnight? I made this a priority.

I dug deep into the internet, researching, and learning all I could about gluten related illnesses. Meanwhile, my guts were now healing as I was doing all I could by eating non-gluten foods. I had now eliminated the antidepressants and the prescription strength vitamins entirely. I felt so much better after 10 months! I wanted to thrive being alive. During this time, I was also noticing that all my research pointed to the fact that hidden gluten lived in almost all foods except vegetables and fruits. At this time, I had a major lightbulb moment! The safest food for me to eat was a whole food, plant-based diet. Now, the fears of eating out, buying food at grocery stores, eating at other people's houses would be greatly reduced when changing to WFPB living.

But how? How could I do this by myself? Initially, I would cry in the aisles at the grocery store because I couldn't figure out what to buy and how to decipher the labels. I then turned to whole food, plant-based support groups on social media. I read as many books as I could find. I realized that I could totally do this! Going plant-based after already being gluten free made a huge difference. I felt so much healthier and had much more energy. The emotional change alone was key! No more fears about getting cross-contaminated with gluten because I knew exactly what to eat and how to prepare foods. I am still learning how much there is to enjoy in the plant-based world. And guess what? I found that I no longer suffered from hypoglycemia.

And then, I noticed that all my inhalers and steroids in my cabinet had expired! What? I had not had an asthma attack in a while. Me, the little girl who wanted new lungs, finally free to live life fully as an adult and with my own daughter. I realized that I hadn't even used them this whole time I had been changing my diet, and especially after cutting out gluten and animal-based foods.

I never knew this could happen. Only once in 2020 did I have to take steroids and my nebulizer during a bout of a bad cold. To be honest, I feel very blessed to have had the celiac diagnosis. Due to this diagnosis, I have dug deeply into the WFPB community, reading various books as they are published, watching documentaries, and following many others on social media. I was driven to learn the truth about food, nutrition advocacy and self-care.

I feel I am truly blessed. I never expected to heal my asthma, IBS, celiac disease, Hashimoto's, hormones, and infertility issues. Even more importantly, my mental health was completely changed by the way I ate. I am free from antidepressants. I no longer suffer from the panic attacks that governed my life nor the depression I endured from a very young age. If I had known earlier, I would have started a whole food, plant-based diet much earlier. It is part of my mission to help others and why I was thrilled to share my story in this book with you.

Today, I consciously choose not to harm my body in any way by the foods that I eat, and I help others through my blog, social media, and consulting others. I am honored to help anyone who is seeking support in changing their health, diet and their life through a whole food, plant-based lifestyle.

Jackie Olmstead

FROM GESTATIONAL DIABETES TO HEALTHY PREGNANCY

VALERIA POPOV

Conditions: Gestational diabetes, overweight, negative body image, sexual insecurity, allergies

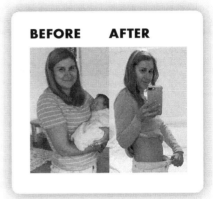

BEFORE   AFTER

Valeria was overweight and had terrible allergies. At age 33 she developed gestational diabetes with her second pregnancy. Valeria was prescribed insulin, and in ever-increasing amounts. Searching for an alternative to injecting herself with insulin, she came across the whole food, plant-based lifestyle. With great trepidation, she switched to a whole plant food lifestyle when she was six months pregnant. It worked wonderfully: In one week her glucose was normal and in two weeks she was off insulin completely. The benefits just keep on coming. Three months after giving birth, she was down 50 pounds. Her allergies had disappeared, and her self-image had vastly improved. There were so many benefits from her plant-based lifestyle, Valeria decided to share the good news by launching a YouTube channel called, The Supercharged Plant-Based Lifestyle.

I have struggled with my body image and my weight since I was 16 years old.

I have tried all kinds of diets. Most of them were unhealthy and I didn't even know it. Many of the diets worked, and I was able to lose weight. But I was never able to stay on a diet. I derailed and gained my weight back. And then some. That part was the most frustrating!

I was overweight, and I hated my body. I was full of allergies, and my skin showed it. I was on allergy medications for many years. I could not look at myself in the mirror. It was too horrible. I could not have sex with my husband without noticing my rolls of fat; It was so embarrassing! You can imagine how "pleasurable" sex was with those thoughts.

Every year, I had seasonal allergies. I was also allergic to dust and had other allergies. I even had weird allergic reactions to water from late spring and early summer showers. I would take Aller-Tec (cetirizine hydrochloride, an over-the-counter antihistamine) every day for 12 years. If I forgot to take it for even one day, I would break out in hives all over my body.

Shopping, which should be an enjoyable activity for a woman, was miserable. Forget about getting a two-piece bathing suit for a vacation! No way! I was constantly restricting myself food-wise, feeling shame and guilt whenever I would eat something that I knew would make me gain weight. I had no confidence and jealousy was continuously driving my thoughts.

Fast forward to my most recent pregnancy when I was diagnosed with gestational diabetes. Insulin was prescribed and the dose kept increasing every week. My doctor could not help me other than to give me more insulin.

I took a class in the hospital on how to deal with gestational diabetes and a couple of nurses taught us what to eat and what to avoid. They advised us to avoid eating fruits. Avoid fruits? After that class, I grew concerned about their teaching against fruits. I always thought fruits were essential during pregnancy.

Around that time, I came across some information online about a plant-based lifestyle and how it helps people with diabetes. There was a Facebook group I came across called Lean and Clean, where I found out about the many benefits of a whole plant food lifestyle. The Lean and Clean Facebook Group was created by Jul Nov, and she had a huge influence on my finding the path to whole food, plant-based living.

I got more curious and started to dig into it more. I had heard people criticize plant-based diets for supposedly being deficient in calcium and protein, claiming we couldn't get all our essential nutrients from plants. (This criticism, I later discovered, was totally false and inaccurate, and may have originated with the meat and dairy industries.) At this point, I was six months into my pregnancy, and I had no other option except insulin shots. So, I decided to give a whole plant food diet a try.

Was I scared? Yes!

I was so brainwashed about the benefits of animal products that this new information about the benefits of a plant-based lifestyle went into me with great resistance. So, I decided to try it for two weeks and see what happens. Besides, I was sick and tired of pricking my fingers after each meal, to the point where I could not prick through my skin any longer because it had gotten so thick and hard from the constant pricking.

In just one week my glucose level was normal and in two weeks I was off insulin!

I was so happy that I didn't need to do insulin shots! I was so relieved that my baby and I were safe!

The remainder of my pregnancy was healthy. I had a fast and easy delivery.

One month postpartum, I went from a weight of 185 pounds to 155 pounds. Three months postpartum, I was down to 136 pounds!

I was now able to enjoy intimate times with my husband. He had my full attention without me worrying about how I looked.

After I experienced the benefits of a plant-based lifestyle, I became not only a true believer but an active advocate for it. I started doing research, joining communities wherever I could, meeting and interacting with other plant-based people in person and online, doing this all around the globe. Searching, reading books, and researching papers, finding and following the best doctors, doing everything I could to plunge into this new, plant-based world.

I found a very simple method that changed the course of my life forever. I pieced together different things that I learned in different places and tried them out. Not only was I healthier than I had ever been, but by using this method I found that it also affected my weight in a very big way. After making some simple changes like going off oil, sugar, salt, and flour, I've lost an additional 20 pounds. It felt amazing. Never in my adult life was I that fit without starving myself. I felt like I gained superpowers!

It was truly powerful to wake up each morning in my new body, step on the scale and see that I am the same skinny person I was yesterday (or even skinnier). It was magical!

Now my confidence is through the roof. My energy is through the roof. My mind is clear and vibrant. Food energizes me. I play with my kids wildly and have tons of energy and fun. I look at myself in the mirror and can't help but wink at myself. I no longer need to take allergy pills. I've gained lean, strong muscles. I am happy and joyful like never before in my life.

Even more important was realizing that the results of what I look like now, and how I feel, are 100% within my power to achieve. I want to recognize that what happened to me was also becoming part of a strong, like-minded community that supported me on my journey. Communities like the National Health Association (NHA) are priceless. If people want results, the first thing I recommend is to join a community.

After so many benefits and so much support from the plant-based community, I decided it was time for me to give back to people. Now it's my turn to share the information that helped me optimize health and weight loss. So, I created a YouTube channel and an online show called, *The Supercharged Plant-Based Lifestyle*. On this show, I share my story and my experiences of weight loss, as well as giving recipes and weight loss strategies that helped me to be where I am today. I also interviewed 30 experts on different topics of healthy living and the power of plants.

Mark Huberman, the president of the National Health Association, and editor of *Health Science* magazine was one of the people I interviewed. I gave away this show for free to people who could benefit from it and from my story. My passion and vision are to support as many people as I can to achieve their optimal health and fitness.

My message to people who are not plant-based now is to try it and see what they might find out. I am pretty sure they will find out that if they have type 2 diabetes, they don't have to shoot insulin for the rest of their lives. (If they have type 1 diabetes, they might be able to greatly reduce their drug dosage.) They might find out that they can get off blood pressure medications within one month, or they might find out that losing weight is much easier than previous experiences. And so much more!

Try it!

What have you got to lose, other than excess weight and medications?

Valeria Popov

FROM DIABETES TO PLANT-BASED TELEHEALTH

ANTHONY MASIELLO

Conditions: Obesity, diabetes, migraines, hypertension, liver problems, psoriasis, eczema, sleep apnea

Anthony Masiello was unhealthy and obese for most of his life. He finally decided to do something about it by switching to a whole food, plant-based lifestyle. In 20 months, he lost 160 pounds and reversed all medical issues, completely transforming his life. Since reclaiming his own health, Anthony has made it his mission to help others do the same. In early 2020, he co-founded Plant-Based TeleHealth, a national telemedicine service focused on the reversal and prevention of chronic disease through a

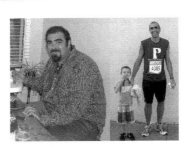

Anthony Masiello –
before & after, with son

whole plant food lifestyle. The goal of Plant-Based TeleHealth is to make lifestyle medicine, rooted in whole food plant-based nutrition, available to everyone. Plant-Based TeleHealth provides medical care via lifestyle medicine and plant-based nutrition. Plant-Based Telehealth physicians are available to provide licensed medical care to patients in all 50 states and Washington D.C. from the comfort and privacy of their home. You can contact Anthony at: **anthony@pbtelehealth.com** *or reach out to:* **https://plantbasedtelehealth.com**

In October of 2005, I felt the pain that started me on this journey, and I remember like it was yesterday. I came home from work and looked through the stack of mail on the counter. I found a letter from an insurance company about a life insurance policy that I had recently applied for. I was a little anxious, because I had issues getting insurance a few years earlier and ended up being put into a higher risk category, which meant I had to pay more for the coverage. I had to pay about 6 times as much as my wife, for the same coverage. It was a bummer, but I paid it and was covered.

I opened the letter, and there it was. Denied. Nothing mentioned about going into another risk category, or follow-up medical assessment, just denied. This company would not sell me a 20-year term life insurance policy. It might as well have said, "No thank you. As much as we would love to take your money every month, your life is not worth it."

In my mind, I immediately translated this into a 20-year death sentence. This huge company, with all the data in the world, ran the numbers and doesn't think I'm going to make it another 20 years. That hit me hard. I can still feel it, being told I had less than 20 years to live, at a stage in life where I should have felt like I was just getting started, with an 18-month-old son, and our second on the way.

As I stood there, 33 years old, on medication for high blood pressure, weighing more than 360 pounds, with a 54-inch waist, I felt depressed and hopeless. Thinking to myself, how did this happen? Why did this happen? I'm not a bad guy. My life isn't so bad. I'm not so unhealthy. Or am I? I did have a few issues that I was dealing with, and a few others that I was admittingly ignoring....

Medical/health issues before:

- Morbidly obese (BMI 45)
- Hypertensive (medicated - TOPROL-XL)
- High cholesterol (214 – unmedicated)
- Liver damage (AST 55, ALT 71, GGT 78)
- Diagnosed with sleep apnea (declined treatment)
- Lifelong migraine headaches (prescribed Imitrex)
- Lifelong eczema on my fingers
- Psoriasis on my neck and head

Looking back, there were lots of good things happening in my life. My wife and I were married and in love, living in our dream home, and starting a family. I had a good job that I enjoyed. We did lots of fun things like snowboarding, biking, and skateboarding. We spent lots of time with friends.

At the same time, there were things that were difficult for me. At 6 feet 4 inches tall, and weighing 360 pounds, it was painful for me to sit in armchairs in the conference rooms at work. I overflowed my seat on airplanes when I had to travel, and I had to ask the flight attendant for the seat belt extension just so I could buckle up. I couldn't shop for clothes in regular stores, everything had to be ordered. I had to buy everything heavy duty from ladders to oversized chairs. I couldn't even weigh myself on a normal bathroom scale!

I shrugged off all of those things with a simple statement. I was a giant. Being both tall and overweight, I somehow justified my being bigger, taller, and wider than everyone else. I'm sure others saw right through that, and I now know this is a classic victim mentality, but at the time it was enough for me to brush it off and not really do anything about it. Until one day at the local carnival.

Late in the summer of 2005, my wife, Cathy, and I were walking around the local church fair. I was carrying my 18-month-old son, Evan, against my chest. We were pointing out the lights, and the rides, with all the bells and sounds of the fair going on in the background. As we walked around a corner,

Evan spotted it. There was Thomas the Train! I don't even remember if it was Thomas or not, but to Evan it didn't matter. He spotted it, and he was excited, and that got me excited for him. We walked closer, and as we approached the ride, I started to pull Evan from my chest to hand him to Cathy, so she could take him on the ride. But, as I did that, he held onto my shirt and pulled. He didn't want to let go, he didn't want to be handed off to my wife, I felt like he wanted me to take him.

The truth is, there was no way I was going to fit on the little train. I didn't even fit on most of the adult rides, how was I ever going to get into that tiny train that was made for kids? The struggle didn't last long at all, probably not more than a few seconds, and Evan was in Cathy's arms and climbing onto the train, getting ready for the ride of his life. As they went through, the attendant asked me to step aside, and wait behind the railing. And there I was, literally standing behind a metal fence, watching, as my wife and son circled the track, giggling, laughing, and having fun.

I stood there, outside the fence, and felt like a bystander. Like an observer of my own life. Unable to do something that I really wanted to be a part of. I thought to myself, "Is this the kind of dad I'm going to be? Is this the kind of husband I am? Is this the kind of life I am going to have?"

I knew the answers to those questions were yes, and I hated that! What I was experiencing, standing outside that ride on that day, was exactly the life that I had created for myself, and I wasn't happy about it at all. When I combined my experience at the fair with all the little annoyances that were starting to add up, and now being denied a 20-year life insurance policy, I was ready to change.

You see, I grew up heavy. I was always the fat kid, and then the big guy. I had tried to lose weight several times throughout my life. Sometimes it worked for a few months, or even a year, and then before I knew it the weight would be back. I was so determined at this point! I wanted to do it and I wanted it to be different. I wanted to be healthy, and I wanted it to last. The only problem was I didn't know what to do. Obviously, I had not yet found anything that had worked for me, but I started anyway.

It was December now, and I was going to make 2006 my year. I set a New Year's resolution to lose 50 pounds in 2006. I immediately gave up sweets and soda. I was going to figure out how to just eat less. I did that for a few months. I didn't eat any sweets, I didn't drink any soda, and I was controlling my portions and keeping myself hungry. And, after three months of doing exactly that, I saw absolutely zero results. I had not lost a single pound! I still had time though, so I kept searching for something that was going to work for me.

In March of 2006, I found it.

While searching Amazon for weight loss books, I came across Dr. Fuhrman's book, *Eat to Live*. I read the description, and it made a lot of sense to me. Eat nutrient dense, whole unprocessed plants, and almost nothing else. I read the reviews, and it seemed to be working for a lot of people. They were getting the results I wanted. I bought the book, read it and changed my diet immediately.

I focused on eating a lot more fruits, vegetables, beans, nuts, and seeds, and at the same time I ate a lot less of everything else. I did not make hard rules in the beginning about the things I would not eat. I really focused on eating more vegetables and fruit and let that crowd out the bad stuff. It was a good plan for me. There were no feelings of failure, and I woke up every day on a mission to eat more healthy vegetables and fruit than I had the day before. And it worked!!

By the time my second son, Henry, was born on May 2, 2006, just 2 months after buying *Eat to Live*, I was already down 30 pounds. I almost couldn't believe it, but I loved it. That was all the motivation I needed to keep pushing.

I continued, eating more and more vegetables, fruits, beans, nuts, and seeds, and cutting out everything else, including oil, breads, flour, sauces, sweeteners, and even pizza. I ate huge salads, and tons of greens. I made big batches of bean chili with mushrooms and kale. I made delicious soups with broccoli and roasted red peppers. I ate everything over steamed spinach, chopped romaine, kale, or other greens, and always with a side of steamed asparagus, broccoli, or brussels sprouts. I snacked on fresh fruit, carrots, and celery. I seriously ate more vegetables and fruit than I ever thought possible, and it was working.

After those first two months, things settled in, and I was losing almost exactly 8 pounds a month. I also started going to see my doctor every two weeks, to track my changes, and to adjust my medications as needed. She started ramping down my blood pressure medication almost immediately, and I noticed that I was experiencing fewer migraine headaches. She was also very impressed with the rate I was losing the weight, and just kept telling me to continue doing what I was doing.

I really liked hearing that. This was a totally different experience than what I was used to. I always dreaded going to see my doctors in the past, because they told me everything that was wrong, tried to get me to go for tests, told me I needed to sleep with creams and gloves on my hands and an oxygen mask on my face, and they tried to start me on medications that I didn't want to take. But not anymore, now my doctor was happy with what I was doing, taking me off medications, and telling me that what I was doing was making me healthy.

By December of 2006, one year into this attempt to lose weight and get healthy, and just 10 months after reading the book *Eat to Live* and changing my diet, my blood pressure was normal without medications. I was no longer experiencing migraine headaches, and I had lost a total of 90 pounds. It was really working, and I couldn't have been happier.

It was the end of the year again, though, and it was time for me to set another New Year's resolution. What was I going to do, other than just continue? This diet was working great. But now, for the first time in my life, I decided that I wanted to start exercising.

It's worth taking a second here, to point out that I lost more than 90 pounds without exercising at all. I mean nothing. I never went for a walk around the block. I never went for a bike ride. I didn't step foot into a gym. nothing, absolutely nothing. I want to make that crystal clear, to highlight the power of the diet changes I made. However, with 90 pounds gone, and my body being healthier than ever, I had energy, lots more energy, more energy than ever. I wanted to do something with it and decided that I was going to start running.

I had never played sports or exercised regularly in my life. I was, at times, physically active, riding bicycles, skateboarding, and snowboarding; but I never exercised regularly. That was about to change. I wanted to start running.

I didn't know what to do, but my wife had a treadmill in the basement, and I went down to give it a try. I started walking. Then, I would run for 30 seconds or so until I lost my breath and go back to walking. I did that for a half hour, every day, and just kept trying to run a little longer each time. I progressed quickly, to the point where I could run a minute, then a quarter mile, then a half mile, then eventually I could run for a full mile. I would warm up, run a mile, take a walk break, and run another. I just continued and the runs got longer, and the walk breaks got shorter, until I could run a few miles in a row.

In March, I signed up to run my first 5k race, and it was the coolest thing. Being out there with everyone hustling around the registration area, signing up, getting bibs, warming up – it was like a swarm of bees all moving in different directions getting ready for the same thing. I couldn't believe that I was a part of it! After that race, I was hooked, and I knew it. I was hooked on a healthy lifestyle that included eating a whole food plant-based diet and running.

I continued progressing with both in 2007. I kept eating more and more vegetables, fruits, beans, nuts, and seeds, and almost nothing else. I also kept increasing my running, by trying to extend my longer runs a little farther and farther every time. Even with adding all this exercise, I continued losing almost exactly 8 pounds a month, every single month, until September 2007 when my weight loss stopped just as suddenly as it began. At that point, I had lost a total of 160 pounds with a new weight of 197. My blood pressure, triglycerides, and cholesterol were all ideal without medication. I was no longer getting migraine headaches, was down 18 inches to a 36-inch waist, and I re-applied and got that life insurance policy, in the preferred category!

On top of that, the peace of mind that I gained is immeasurable. Knowing that I am truly healthy is priceless. Knowing that I am going to be an active part of my family's lives for a very long time means the world to me.

Medical/health issues after:

- ~~Morbidly obese (BMI 45)~~ ➡ **BMI 24**
- ~~Hypertensive (medicated - TOPROL-XL)~~ ➡ **Blood pressure ideal (115/71)**
- ~~High cholesterol (214 – unmedicated)~~ ➡ **Cholesterol ideal (128)**
- ~~Liver damage (AST 55, ALT 71, GGT 78)~~ ➡ **Liver tests ideal (29, 23, 31)**
- ~~Diagnosed with sleep apnea (declined treatment)~~ ➡ **No more sleep apnea**
- ~~Lifelong migraine headaches (prescribed Imitrex)~~ ➡ **No more headaches**
- ~~Lifelong eczema on my fingers~~ ➡ **No more eczema**
- ~~Psoriasis on my neck and head~~ ➡ **No more psoriasis**

My life is better in every way. All the activities I enjoyed doing growing up (snowboarding, skateboarding, riding motorcycles, bicycling, etc.) are easier and more fun than ever. I have new healthy activities that my family and I do together, like running, playing basketball, and hiking all over the country.

The self confidence that I have gained through the process of truly taking care of myself has changed my life so much more than any of these physical changes. I'm a better friend, husband, father, and member of society than I have ever been. Professionally, I went from being a shy person who hesitated to speak in most situations to becoming an outspoken leader who can align teams on strategy and deliver outstanding results.

I couldn't be more happy or proud to live this lifestyle with my wife and my sons, Evan, and Henry, who are now 14 and 12 years old. They are proud to visit the doctor once a year for a wellness checkup and hear the doctor say the same thing every time "Oh, the healthy family is here."

We literally feel good and have fun every day, and we get to go on some amazing adventures together. The feelings I get from truly living life, the way that we do that now as a family, being able to help others, is beyond my wildest dreams. There is nothing that would ever make me want to give that up.

The best advice I can give to someone thinking about making a change for themselves is - do it! I promise that if you adopt and commit to figuring out how to make this lifestyle work, you will get the results that you are looking for, and you will be happy you did it.

That's not to say that it will be easy. It will be difficult in the beginning as you transition, but the longer you stick with it, the easier it gets, and eventually it will become your preferred way of living and eating. I've seen it happen so many times. I look forward to seeing so many more of these life transformations.

You can do it!

Anthony Masiello

FOR MY HEALTH, FOR MY GOALS, FOR MY LIFE

MARY SNYDER

Conditions: Obesity, heart disease, fatigue, toenail fungus

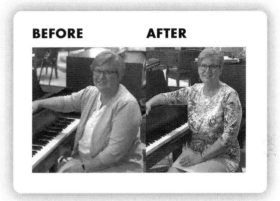

BEFORE   AFTER

Mary Snyder grew up on a small farm in Iowa with her two older brothers. She is currently a school counselor near Des Moines, Iowa having spent over 35 years in the field of education. In 2013, Mary published a book titled "Teachable Moments" about her work with students. She is working on a new book about her experiences growing up on the farm, including stories about her first paid job of catching nightcrawlers for the local bait shop. Mary's mother still lives on that farm. Mary can be reached at m02snyder@gmail.com.

You don't have to look far to notice the growing waistline of the public. The resulting weight loss programs with creative marketing strategies are growing, too. We have plenty of food available but deciding what and how much to eat is becoming an industry unto itself. In the end, everyone makes their own choices and does what works for them. I found what works for me. This is my story.

I have struggled with weight for most of my life. From middle school onward I've been near the top end of the weight and height chart. There were periods of time when it wasn't a problem, but I am not naturally slender and any weight I would lose always found its way back to me and then some.

Over time, I put a lot of money and effort into losing extra pounds. I tried Weight Watchers, LA Weight Loss, Medi-Fast, gym memberships, personal trainers and whatever programs were the flavor of the day. Everything worked for a while, until it didn't. But counting calories, tracking meals or other requirements eventually became too much work and the cycle would start all over again.

By the time I had reached my early 50's, my age was starting to catch up with me. While there are many benefits to being active, the numbers on the scale weren't as low as they had been in younger years, no matter how much I exercised or how I ate.

Then a difficult period in my life prompted a great deal of emotional eating. For some years, my typical lunch consisted of two slices of convenience store pizza (Canadian bacon if available), a bag of baked potato chips and 20 ounces of Diet Dr. Pepper Cherry. I would purchase another 20 ounces of soda for the afternoon. Sometimes that menu was repeated for supper. I just didn't have the energy to care about anything, which was obvious from numbers on the scale.

One day, a new pain began in the heel of my right foot. It hurt a lot. It was difficult to walk, each step felt like I was stepping down on a hot dagger. I figured it was due to my increasing weight. A fungus had also crept into my right toenail. My physical activity came to a screeching halt and my typically busy workday was spent seated as much as possible.

Going to the doctor was something I only did every other year unless I was sick. I know part of my hesitation involved stepping on the scale, but my foot was so painful that I finally made an appointment. The physician's assistant didn't seem too concerned and said I probably had plantar fasciitis and showed me how to wrap my foot and gave me exercises to do. This helped, but not much. I was given the impression that it would eventually go away.

Many months later, I was looking forward to a wellness retreat in California and decided to see a podiatrist, hoping there was something more to be done about the pain, so I could enjoy the trip. A few injections later and I had a new lease on life.

Unfortunately, my food choices coupled with inactivity had caused my weight to explode. My standard height of 5' 8½" was slowly shrinking, but my usual weight of 160 had ballooned to 240! I did this to myself. I could blame many things and I had lots of excuses, but it came down to the choices of what I ate and how much I put into my body.

I wasn't just fat, I was obese. I was bloated. My skin looked unhealthy. Even my hair was limp. I couldn't stand to look at myself in the mirror. My body was screaming for help, and I was too tired and heavy to do anything about it.

Every season, I bought larger sizes of clothing and put them in laundry baskets around my bedroom. Eventually another season would roll around and I'd be so disgusted that I had to go shopping again. I refused to get rid of the smaller clothes because it felt like giving up. I was convinced I'd wear those sizes again, but my bedroom became steadily smaller as my clothing became steadily larger.

In July of 2017 I noticed I couldn't sing a phrase without catching my breath. I love to sing so this problem really caught my attention. I noticed other issues. There was a mild pain in my sternum, and my regular donations to the local blood bank were taking increasingly longer, up to 25 minutes to fill a pint bag. I went back to the doctor who sent me to see a cardiologist. He ran all sorts of tests which came back fine, but he said "If you don't lose the weight then in about five years, we're going to be seeing a lot of each other. Follow a Mediterranean diet, use olive oil and eat lean protein."

I figured I had some time before I needed to get serious about my health, but I did make a half-hearted attempt to follow his suggestions. The sternum pain eventually went away but the shortness of breath lingered.

One evening in late October 2018 I was watching TV and felt a tickle in my chest. It didn't hurt, but it was annoying. It went away, then came back a little stronger. This went on for about an hour and I considered going to Urgent Care, but it was closed, so I'd have to go to the ER. I felt fine otherwise: steady pulse, no sweating, no other pain, only this strange random tickle in my left chest. I didn't want to go to the ER, so I did what many people do in this situation and just went to bed.

My thinking was that I would feel better once I laid down. Wrong. That made it worse. I finally propped myself up with pillows to a point where I was comfortable and had started to relax when I wondered if I should leave a note on the kitchen table in case I didn't wake up in the morning. But that meant I'd have to go through the hassle of getting comfortable again, so I decided to take my chances and stay in bed. I didn't think I would die overnight, but it was odd to consider the possibility.

Much to my relief I woke up the next morning bright and early like normal. I stayed in bed for a while taking stock of how I was feeling. The tickle was still there but I started thinking about my health. I wasn't afraid of dying, but I wanted to LIVE. I didn't want to be the fat lady who watched everyone else enjoy their lives while I sat with chest pain, eating myself to death. Was it only one year ago when the cardiologist said I might have problems in five years? Did I do five years of damage in twelve months?

Had I run out of time?

While trying not to panic about this, a phrase went through my head that I had heard earlier "Being fat is hard. Losing weight is hard. Pick your hard."

I knew about being fat and I knew about losing weight. Both were hard, but only one offered the life I wanted for myself. I knew what didn't work, but there had to be something that did work. So, in the quiet of that morning, grateful to be alive, an internal switch flipped, and I picked my hard. I made the decision to not just lose the weight, but to gain back my health. This was in my control.

I knew there was not a canned program out there that would work for me. Those programs might work well for others, but I needed to be accountable to myself, not to the lady who read my food journal or tracked my weight or sold me snacks made in a food lab. I needed to be accountable to the lady who looked at me in the mirror every day. The tickle lasted for about a week, but I never did find out what was causing it.

I got out of bed that morning and started looking online for ideas when I stumbled onto *Bright Line Eating* by Susan Pierce Thompson. It looked interesting. The Bright Lines were four things that you absolutely had to commit to follow. No sugar. No flour. No eating between meals and watch quantities by weighing your food. This sounded strict but clear cut. However, watching quantities meant measuring and I didn't think I would stick to that, so I kept looking.

While watching a video of Susan Pierce Thompson, she mentioned that she was asked to be on a panel by someone named Jon McMahon. He was doing nine hour-long interviews with experts about weight loss and nutrition, one interview per day for nine days. No cost. Jon was about my age, but much heavier and diabetic. Like me, he knew he had to make some changes. I signed up to watch the interviews. They were interesting and talked a lot about overall health, nutrition, and the science behind food. He referenced physicians like Dr. Caldwell Esseslstyn, Dr. Colin Campbell, and many others. One of the things I heard mentioned frequently in these interviews was a Netflix documentary, also on YouTube, called *Forks Over Knives*. I watched it and I was hooked.

The name *Forks Over Knives* refers to watching what is on your fork to keep you away from the knife of heart surgery and other health problems. It talked about the dangers of sugar, flour, and unhealthy fats which didn't surprise me, but it also talked about the dangers of dairy, red meat and other animal products. I grew up on a small Iowa farm and we ate what we grew. What we grew was a large vegetable garden as well as dairy cows, cattle, pigs and chickens. This got me thinking.

I had chores on the farm. I had to help weed the garden and feed the animals. We fed them grain and let them loose in the pasture. Never once did we feed our animals meat or expect them to stalk prey for food. Thinking more about this, I realized all the large animals like elephants and gorillas, among others, don't eat meat or hunt for their meals. They eat plants. They don't drink milk after being weaned, but they still get strong. So why do we have to eat the animals when the animals are eating plants? Can we just skip the animals and eat plants ourselves?

The animals that do eat meat are not the animals that we eat. The local grocer doesn't offer Lion Loins or Cheetah Chops at the meat counter, right? It all seems counterintuitive. I know there are ethical and environmental reasons people choose to avoid animal products and I respect those reasons, but the one that really got my attention was making the connection of what we fed or didn't feed our animals on the farm.

The documentary Forks Over Knives got my attention in a way like nothing else did. The primary message of the documentary is to follow a whole food, plant-based lifestyle, with no oil, minimal salt, and eat until you are full. Avoid highly processed foods and don't eat meat, fish, dairy, or any other animal products. Examples of whole foods would be having an orange instead of orange juice or having a potato instead of French fries. Examples of plants are too numerous to mention.

I could do this. By now it was mid-November 2018 and I decided to try it for one week. I finished off the rotisserie chicken, yogurt, eggs, and butter that were in my fridge. I changed my breakfast from two poached eggs on toast, to oatmeal topped with blueberries and cinnamon. The convenience store lunch was replaced by a spinach salad with walnuts, tofu, and other toppings from home. My dinner shifted from Chinese take-out, a sandwich of deli meats, or whatever else looked good at the meat counter to sweet potatoes, steamed broccoli, cauliflower, and a handful of black beans.

At the end of the week, I looked less bloated. I decided to go another week. Then another. Two months later, I had lost almost 20 pounds. In six months, I lost almost 60 pounds! I gave away laundry baskets of clothing, and freezer bags of meat and ice cream. The toenail fungus went away. My blood donations took six minutes, and I could once again sing long phrases of my solo at Easter services without needing to catch my breath.

I haven't looked back once.

My new family doctor isn't so sure about my food choices, but she can't argue with my lab work, most of which is moving in the right direction. People I eat with notice my colorful meals and say 'wow, that looks healthy'. I notice how brown their meals look. My taste buds have changed. Maybe I could force myself to eat meat, but it doesn't even look good anymore. The bonus of it not being appealing means that no will power is involved, so I don't need to talk myself out of eating something that I really don't want to eat.

My gut has changed, too. One well-meaning friend invited me to a brunch where she served coffee cake and French toast. I ate some and about 20 minutes later my stomach revolted violently. I used to eat cheese by the handful, but now it looks greasy, and the crackers that I would munch on until the box was empty now are tasteless. My new favorite snack is grapes, which I eat like I used to eat M&M's.

At a recent cook out of burgers and brats, I brought a marinated portabella mushroom and asked the grill master to put it on the grill. He did, and it tasted wonderful in a bun with condiments. At a recent office potluck, I wasn't even tempted to eat what was there, except for the vegetable platter and bowl of fruit that was left when the other bowls were empty. Everything on the serving tables looked brown: wings, beef tips, chips, brownies, cookies, and other brown items. I got a few funny looks as I ate my salad with spinach, grilled mushrooms, peppers, tofu, sprouts, tomatoes, and black beans topped off with a drizzle of balsamic vinegar, and a juicy peach for dessert. I enjoyed my meal, and they may have enjoyed theirs, though some co-workers commented that they felt sluggish and were ready for a nap. I remember having that sluggish feeling, but it doesn't happen anymore!

Once in a while, I wonder if this is all worth it. Not many other people I know follow this way of eating, and sometimes it's a hassle. It's difficult to be at a function and just drink coffee because there's nothing there that I would choose to eat, or to be traveling and struggle with meal choices while on the road. This quote helps me: "If you quit now, you'll be back to where you first started; when you first started you were desperate to be where you are now."

People tell me I look healthy. I feel so much better but I'm a work in progress. I do moderate exercise on a treadmill, lift weights, and occasionally go to yoga classes. The most consistent exercise I get is walking my dog. I still have more weight to lose but I'm eating whole foods and sticking with plant-based foods.

For my health. For my goals. For my life.

Here are my health numbers. They have improved amazingly:

MARY SNYDER LAB WORK	2015	2017	2019	2020
Blood pressure		142/80	110/71	100/65
Hemoglobin	13.3	11.9	13.4	14.1
Triglycerides	48	51	100	69
Total Cholesterol	261	247	213	200
LDL	167	142	131	125
HDL	84	95	62	61

Mary Snyder

FROM ALMOST A FINGER AMPUTEE TO ACCOMPLISHED ARTIST

DAVID & GLENDA BRIDGES

Conditions: Lupus, scleroderma, Sjogren's disease, necrotizing fasciitis, arthritis, allergies, seizures

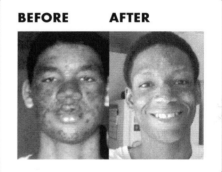

BEFORE AFTER

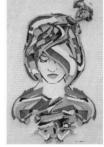

David's artwork bought by Dan Purjes

*David Bridges and his mother, Glenda, want to share their story of his amazing disease reversal as a beacon of hope to all those who are unwell. David says, "Never give up!" He was sick for so many years with lupus and other diseases, that he never thought there would be a solution. At the height of his diseases, David was intubated in a hospital in Los Angeles. Doctors there recommended amputation of several fingertips because they could not control his infections. Glenda refused to give permission for the amputations. Fortunately, she met Dr. Brooke Goldner, who had reversed **lupus and other** diseases in her own body. Dr. Goldner, whose story is elsewhere in this book, guided David to a whole food, plant-based lifestyle. That reversed his diseases in a few months. No amputations needed! David was able to live a normal life and resume his passion as an artist. He was one of the first people who reversed autoimmune disease met by Dan Purjes, the co-author of this book. That meeting became the seed for the creation of this book. Dan bought one of David's artworks as a memento of that significant moment. David has now had gallery shows for his artwork in Los Angeles.*

GLENDA BRIDGES TELLS THE STORY

My son, David, was heavily sedated in a Los Angeles hospital bed with tubes running in and out of his body. He had lupus and other diseases that often accompany lupus. The infections on his leg and fingers were so bad, so out of control, that doctors advised amputation of several fingers and possibly a leg. They were afraid gangrene might set in. I was in anguish. I refused to give permission to cut off my son's leg and fingers.

How could I do that to my son?

A while later, I met Dr. Brooke Goldner[1] who once had lupus herself, the same disease that was ravaging my son's body. Dr. Goldner described how she had reversed her lupus completely by converting to a whole food, plant-based diet. She never had a relapse in the many years since.

I asked her to help my son. She guided David to adopt this lifestyle. Today, David is completely healed. He does not have lupus or any of the other diseases that accompanied it. He has no symptoms. He is off all medications and has no biomarkers for the diseases. He has all his fingers and legs. And he is living a normal, healthy life, creating his unique three-dimensional paintings, and doing other work and activities.

It had been fifteen long, hard years of wondering how to gain control of David's health. My son had multiple medical conditions before the two of us learned of this lifestyle change that worked miracles for his diseases and restored him to full health.

When David was 15 years old, he developed strep throat that he caught from a teacher who came to school sick with that disease. I took David to a doctor who, after examining him, asked if David was allergic to penicillin. We told the doctor that David had never taken the medication before, so we were unsure if he would have any allergic reactions. The doctor swabbed David's mouth and concluded that he was fine to take the drug.

He wasn't. Little did we know that after David took the medication his body would experience severe allergic reactions. These ranged from a simple nosebleed to a temperature of 106, from severely swollen hands and feet to a horrible rash, a butterfly rash, that went across his face and chest. He also had other terrible symptoms such as arthritis, that caused terrible pain in his joints, and infections on his hands and legs, and even his face. Pus would come out of the infections, including from his face.

There were several diagnostic tests that were conducted on David that year. The diagnostic results showed that David had Systemic Lupus Erythematosus (SLE), Scleroderma, and Sjogren's diseases. The version of lupus that David had was cutaneous lupus, which created lesions and infections of the skin. All these diseases are autoimmune diseases in which the body's own immune system attacks its organs and tissues, as though they are foreign.

When David turned 21, his ankles became very swollen during the summer months. He was on a cancer chemotherapy drug called Methotrexate, which like other cancer chemotherapy drugs, suppresses and weakens the immune system. This is the standard treatment for many autoimmune diseases — cancer chemotherapy drugs that weaken the immune system, so it does not attack its own body. Of course, a weaker immune system often leads to other ailments, and cancer chemotherapy drugs have very severe side effects.

David's swollen ankles made any type of walking very difficult and painful. One night he got up to go to the bathroom and scratched his right leg against the metal bed in the apartment. It didn't feel like it cut through the skin, so he went back to bed. The next day he saw a tiny scar on his leg, barely noticeable. He thought nothing of it. His swollen ankles were the visible problem we were concerned about. His feet were elevated for about two days while he was confined to bed.

In those two days, while relatives were visiting us, a flesh-eating bacterium had infected the scar and traveled from the top of his foot to just below the knee cap. The doctors referred to it as necrotizing fasciitis in the leg, an infection that spreads very rapidly, killing tissue and muscles as it spreads. About 30% of people who get necrotizing fasciitis die.

The rest of the story could be very long and drawn out. Here is the short version: David spent four months in seven different hospitals. During this time, he had a seizure and was placed on seizure medication (Dilantin), which in turn, caused the skin on his face to slough off. The skin fell off his face, and the layers underneath were exposed as though he was a burn victim.

David spent a lot of time in the ICU. Doctors cut the bacteria out from his leg. It took three surgeries to secure a skin graft to his right leg. The doctors thought the procedure would be problematic because skin grafts usually don't take in individuals with autoimmune conditions, but the procedure was a success.

After three months in hospitals, he was moved to a rehabilitation hospital. He spent a month in rehab gaining strength back in his arms and learning how to walk again. When someone hasn't walked in months, their legs atrophy. The circulation to the feet is all but gone. After spending a month in the rehab hospital, David emerged through the sliding doors using a walker, feeling the wind from a breeze outside for the first time in a long time. He would spend the next year at home, rehabilitating his legs. He recovered well enough to continue his schooling the following summer.

Seven years later, at age 28, David came down with Scleroderma. This disease attacks and constricts circulation in the body. Fingers and toes are usually affected the most, because the blood vessels inside them are small and they are furthest from the heart. The lack of circulation caused an infection in his fingers. He was taking medication to fight off the infection. He was also taking pain medication because once an infection that gets under the skin grows it causes an intense amount of pressure in the finger, and in the entire hand.

He started taking Vicodin and threw up three meals in one day. The next morning, he stopped taking the pain medication, but he felt immensely sick. As the infections worsened, and circulation to his fingers was cut off, the doctors recommended amputating several fingertips to prevent gangrene from setting in. I adamantly refused to allow that.

Glenda Bridges

DAVID CONTINUES THE STORY

In that hospital, my whole body felt weak, my energy was totally gone. My back felt like it was out. For three days, I could only sit up to eat. Then I would go back and rest. My back was too weak to hold my weight for very long.

I don't know why, but at the time there in the hospital, there were a multitude of symptoms happening. One after the other. The most painful was the infection in my fingers. At times, the infection would cut off circulation to the fingers. The doctor told me it was like having frostbite in the fingers. He was afraid that eventually gangrene would develop, and my fingers would have to be amputated. I'm an artist. That's one of the worst things that could happen.

Other symptoms that hit me included open sores on my face and fingers, a large rash on my chest, nerve pain in my lower back and sores inside of my mouth. I had Systemic Lupus and Scleroderma. I had at one point a flesh-eating bacterium in my leg. When that happened, there was talk of possibly having to amputate the leg.

My body, mind and soul had come to the lowest place of my existence.

Despite all these symptoms, the pain and suffering; it was good that I went through this, because it brought me to where I met an angel called Doctor "G," That was Brooke Goldner, M.D., who had lupus herself as a teenager and as a young woman, but then reversed it and several other diseases by converting to a whole food, plant-based diet.

My mother first met Dr. G at a continuing medical education course. My mother works at a mental health clinic. All healthcare professionals are required to take continuing medical education courses, often taught by physicians, to maintain their professional status. Dr. G was teaching the course my mother was taking. Dr. G mentioned that she once had lupus and other related diseases but had reversed them entirely through diet. My mother went right up to her after the course lecture and asked her to help me with my lupus. And she did!

Or rather she did, partly. I adopted Dr. G.'s whole foods, plant-based diet protocol, but only half-heartedly. I ate better, and I felt better, but I also continued to eat inflammatory foods that hindered reversal of my diseases. I did this for two years and experienced some good results. My energy returned, the pains were less, and I was feeling better, but I was not yet healed. I continued to eat some animal-based foods and processed foods.

Sometime later, I attended a talk given by Dr. G in which she explained how the whole foods, plant-based diet had reversed her chronic diseases: lupus, anticardiolipin, and nephritis (kidney disease). She stressed how important it was to adhere to the diet completely to obtain the maximum, optimal results. She emphasized that a partial approach would not fully reverse disease. I then decided to go all in, become fully plant based eating only whole plant foods.

Almost three years have passed since I went all in and adopted a whole food, plant-based diet whole-heartedly. I am feeling better than I ever have in the past sixteen years. It is amazing to me how fast my body is healing itself, and how good I feel.

I notice this in many ways. My platelets clot much faster, and bruises only last a short while. I have no residual symptoms of any kind. There is some joint disfigurement in my fingers from the infections and diseases I suffered, but there are no on-going symptoms of any kind. When I was on chemotherapy drugs and other drugs, they caused my hair to fall out, made me nauseous, and caused other horrible side effects. Now, my hair has grown back, I feel great, and there are no flare ups or other problems. I have been eating this healthy way for a long time.

I am off all medications. All of them. It's like I was never sick.

I don't miss those bad food choices. The whole foods, plant-based lifestyle is the only way to LIVE.

David Bridges

---

[1] Dr. Brooke Goldner's own battle with lupus can be found elsewhere in this book.

FROM HOT MESS TO COOL MAMA

JACKIE LOPEZ

Conditions: Obesity, alcoholism, food addiction, infertility, high cholesterol, hypertension, angina, heart disease, allergies, sinusitis, ear infections, hearing problems, acne, menstrual problems, sexual insecurity

Jackie Lopez struggled with weight from an early age. She began suffering with more and more diseases. By the time she was a teenager, she had a host of ailments. By the time she was 20, she was on a downward spiral of food addiction and alcoholism. By the time she was 25, she was married and a size 18 in clothes, up from a size 4. She also added many other health problems to her roster, including infertility. Jackie found her way to a whole plant food lifestyle and all her ailments reversed in just a few months. Jackie says, "It seems like I became a new person overnight!" Now, Jackie wants to share the bounty of her new life and health with all those still suffering needlessly.

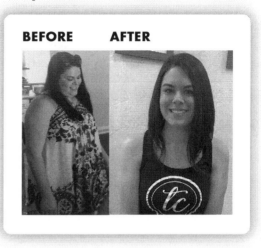

BEFORE   AFTER

Food has always been an experience for me. Growing up in the south with parents who loved to experiment with new foods and refine old favorites left a lasting impression on my life. Trying new recipes (and new restaurants) was always an exciting and happy time for my family. Everything from shopping for the ingredients to the final taste test and presentation was a total thrill. I loved it.

I know that my parents, like lots of other parents, did the best they could with the information they were given when it came to food. Unfortunately, the information they were given was industry-funded and disease-promoting. What my parents had been taught about food was reinforced by my public-school education. I vividly remember sitting in health classes, salivating while my teachers used colorful charts and diagrams to teach about nutrition and a "balanced" diet. I was tantalized by the cartoon pictures of the foods they were promoting meat, cheese, milk, eggs, bread, and pasta. I remember fruits and vegetables being much less emphasized.

As a result of all this, I struggled with my weight from a young age. I was never the heaviest in my class, but I was always heavy enough to know I was different. And always heavy enough to hate it.

In addition to a mainstream diet consisting of lots of meat, dairy, and processed foods, I developed bad snacking habits as an adolescent. The seed of these habits was present when I was very young. I remember my aunt referring to me as a "bottomless pit." She was right. I always felt an insatiable desire to gorge myself on whatever was in front of me until I was completely stuffed. It didn't matter what it was. If I wanted it, I wanted ALL of it, and then some. I remember other people's houses as always having the best snacks!

By the time I was a teenager, I struggled not only with my weight, but with a host of other supposedly "normal" conditions including chronic sinus and ear infections, seasonal allergies, hormonal acne, and terribly painful menstrual periods that were heavy, irregular, and often lasted longer than they should have. I understand now that these conditions were common, but they were NOT normal.

My weight had taken a serious toll on my self-esteem by the time I reached high school. That is when I embarked on my first low-carb diet and exercise regimen. I did my own research at age fourteen to come up with the low-carb diet and exercise program. I lost twenty-three pounds in two months. I was so proud of myself! My confidence was greatly boosted.

Over the six years that followed, I gained and lost the same fifteen to twenty pounds once every year or two, but it seemed to be all I could do to maintain any semblance of health or a body in which I could feel relatively confident. I say "relatively" confident because, no matter how much weight I ever lost, I was never totally comfortable. I was always the girl fidgeting with my clothes or holding couch pillows on my lap to hide my stomach.

Food was both an old friend and an enemy to me, and I didn't know how to reconcile my passion for food with my desire to live a healthy, happy life. It seemed impossible. Still, though, I was at least confident that I always knew how to lose the weight: low-carb dieting, strenuous exercise, and copious amounts of self-control. This worked well for me. Until it didn't.

At age twenty, I found myself rapidly descending a spiral of alcoholism and food addiction, triggered by a series of difficult circumstances, and for which I was primed by a lifetime of addictive binge-eating patterns. I completely lost my will to exercise or control my portions. I never experienced enough will-power to return to low-carb dieting again; I was totally pulled under by addiction.

I ate fast food or restaurant food all day, almost every day during this time. At night, I would eat, then binge drink and eat again. This period lasted for about a year-and-a-half. Then I met my husband, and we got married seven months later, four days after my twenty-second birthday.

I spent the first three years of my marriage still wrestling with alcohol and food addiction. By my twenty-fifth birthday in 2016, I had gained more than eighty pounds, landing me at 213 pounds. I had gone from a strong, fit size four to a size sixteen/eighteen.

I had high cholesterol, chest pains, and blood pressure spikes as high as 154/104. I also experienced chronic ear congestion that caused several very painful ear infections. I had tubes placed in my eardrums for a time to drain the fluid, but it was thick like glue and had to be suctioned out, despite which I still suffered a substantial amount of hearing loss. And to top it all off, I was infertile. This was a devastating blow as I had always longed to have children.

I started crying out to God about my alcohol addiction and my health. I was able to stop habitually drinking in 2017. I also began to see breadcrumbs of information in my life leading me toward a plant-based diet. I had one vegan friend, and my husband and I used to teasingly ask him questions like, "But where do you get your protein?" (I laugh now at how ignorant we were.)

Despite my aversion to the thought of giving up all the foods I had grown up eating, I felt more and more drawn to the plant-based diet as time passed. I spent a lot of time learning about the benefits of plant-based eating, listening to people's health-transformation testimonies, and looking for new recipes to try. By 2018, I knew that the plant-based lifestyle was the one to restore my health, but I really dug my heels in hard. I continued to submit to the powerful pull of addiction by pounding down fast food for breakfast, lunch, and dinner.

My husband traveled a lot for work at the time, so it was easy for both of us to justify eating out, since we couldn't eat at home together anyway. Our marriage and my ability to be at ease with him was greatly impacted by my weight; I was unable to be comfortable with intimacy at all. He often shared with me that he didn't feel like I loved him, and I feared that, because of my weight, he didn't love me either. Our relationship suffered.

In the spring of 2018, I gave dieting and strenuous exercise a final go. I hired a trainer and lost twenty pounds, then yo-yoed back and forth within those twenty pounds for a few months. Finally, after a few more health scares in the summer, I switched completely to a plant-based diet on August 10, 2018, a day I'll always remember as a major defining moment in my life.

Looking back at the few months that followed, it seems like I became a new person overnight. I lost sixty-two pounds in five months without exercising at all, landing me at 131 pounds. My LDL cholesterol dropped sixty-two points in just a couple of months, and my blood pressure went down to about 105/70. Astonishingly, my ear congestion cleared up and my hearing loss reversed.

My seasonal allergies even went away! Within a few months I realized that, for the first time in my life, I had perfectly regular menstrual periods that I could track and predict.

I conceived a child in October of 2019 after more than four years of infertility!

It seems like I experience more and more new benefits of the plant-based diet the longer that it's a part of my life. For the first time in my life, I'm comfortable with how I look, and I don't feel the need to obsess over the number on the scale. My relationship with my husband is wonderful now, and he even jumped on board with plant-based eating after a few months!

I feel light and unencumbered and can enjoy activities without feeling worn out from improperly fueling my body. The list goes on and on.

It is interesting how it seems like all the people I envied when I was young because they were smaller than me are getting bigger and sicker (and blaming age for it) while I become leaner and healthier! I want to share the benefits of plant-based eating with everyone I know. I want everyone to experience the power of reversing years of discomfort with simple dietary changes. The most exciting part is that a healthy diet doesn't have to be boring!

After all I've been through, food is still an experience that I love and is no longer an enemy for me. My husband and I love trying new recipes and making plant-based versions of old favorites. It's fun to watch people's faces when they try our food and then find out it is plant-based! I have a healthy lifestyle that I can enjoy, and I'm so thankful for it. It is overwhelming!

I want people everywhere to know that they can eat this way and enjoy it. I would have never thought it possible, but now that I've experienced the benefits for myself, I'll never go back to my old ways.

A plant-based life is life for me.

Jackie Lopez

TERMINAL CANCER... 30 YEARS AGO
GLENN SABIN

Condition: Chronic Lymphocytic Leukemia (CLL)

In 1991, Glenn Sabin, a 28-year-old newlywed, was diagnosed with chronic lymphocytic leukemia (CLL), a form of leukemia doctors termed "uniformly fatal." Treatments could ease his discomfort, but there was no conventional cure. He was told he had only a few months left to live.

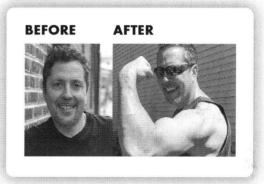

That was 30 years ago. Although he continued to consult with doctors, Glenn made a monumental decision: he would become his own health advocate. While he continued to "watch and wait," as suggested by his physicians, Glenn would figure out how to stay alive. Glenn began his own medically monitored and carefully researched lifestyle changes. He would conduct his own single patient clinical trial. He would become an "n of 1," which is the title of the book he wrote. Today, 30 years later, Glenn is not only living, but thriving. A 2012 biopsy at Harvard Medical confirmed that his bone marrow contains no leukemic cells. His case is now part of the medical literature. Visit **www.glennsabin.com** *and find his book, "n of 1," on Amazon.* **@GlennSabin**

In the fall of 1991, at the age of 28, a routine physical with my primary care physician swiftly changed from its predictable pattern and transformed into a shocking diagnosis of Chronic Lymphocytic Leukemia (CLL).

I was given a dire prognosis: Only six months to live.

That was 30 years ago.

Bruce R. Kressel, MD, a hematologist now associated with the Johns Hopkins system, confirmed the CLL diagnosis via bone marrow biopsy. Apparently, I'd had the disease for some time; my spleen was significantly enlarged. A normal spleen weighs about two-and-a-half pounds. Mine was seven pounds, infiltrated by five pounds of leukemic cells. Two months later, I underwent a splenectomy, a removal of the spleen, to debulk the tumor burden.

PROGNOSIS AND TREATMENT OPTIONS

After recovering from the splenectomy, I sat down with my hematologist to discuss my prognosis and options for treatment. Given my age, he suggested

I obtain a second opinion from a major cancer center. It was arranged and carried out with Lee M. Nadler, MD, a leading CLL clinician investigator at Harvard's Dana-Farber Cancer Institute. I was offered two choices: watchful waiting or bone marrow transplant.

The year 1991 had ushered in a shift in the standard of care from an immediate cocktail of chemotherapeutics to the option of watchful waiting, basically observing the course of disease. The theory was, *when* the disease made a more aggressive move, it would *then* receive a violent assault in the form of multiple chemotherapy agents and steroids.

At that time, bone marrow transplants were essentially experimental options as potentially curative interventions, carrying with them the risk associated with graft-versus-host disease, and a 20% mortality rate. My siblings had their blood tested, but since none matched, allogeneic transplant was ruled out. For reasons I do not recall, we never looked at the marrow registry.

That left the option of an autologous bone marrow transplant — removing some affected bone marrow with biopsy needles, after which my entire immune system would be wiped out with high dose chemo and radiation therapy; my marrow would be eliminated; I would be isolated for an extended period of time. Once the marrow was destroyed, my own 'cleaned' marrow would be reintroduced into my system and stimulated to repopulate. Furthermore, I would be rendered sterile and must bank sperm if I wanted children.

HARD CHOICES

CLL is an older person's disease. I was in my late twenties, newly married, at the prime of life. I was told my condition was terminal, but that I could live a number of years by managing the disease with various interventions, as needed. A palliative approach.

But how could I, a forward-leaning, type A man get comfortable with the two options? Watchful waiting seemed incredibly passive, essentially a sitting duck. The bone marrow transplant appeared incredibly invasive. And there was that 20% mortality rate, too.

Ultimately, I chose neither option and went with what I call 'proactive observation'. I would not simply wait for the other shoe to drop. I would learn what I had to do to become the center of my own healing, playing a meaningful role in the management of disease. After all, I was told that the science of CLL was evolving quickly; apparently new cures were on the horizon. Perhaps I could hold my disease at bay until a curative intervention became available?

BECOMING EMPOWERED

I shared my preferred care approach with my oncology team and asked important questions. What proactive measures could I take to become more involved in my own care? What lifestyle change might positively impact my immune function, or possibly alter the biology of the CLL?

There was unanimity in their response: Nothing I could do would positively affect the course of disease. The leukemia was caused by a genetic malfunction; it was not my fault; diet and exercise would make no difference; I should focus on trying to live the best life I could.

Soon I would understand that my oncology team was not all that interested, or trained, in nutrition and other lifestyle approaches to cancer care. At the time of my diagnosis, the literature was largely void of studies showing the benefit of diet, physical activity, and stress reduction on helping to prevent disease, let alone to control its growth, or to better ensure long-term survivorship. It was incredibly discouraging that my well-regarded oncology team saw zero value in the behavioral change I planned to investigate. I decided to look for others who could support me.

EARLIEST DAYS OF INTEGRATIVE ONCOLOGY

My diagnosis, in 1991, came a dozen years before the founding of the Society for Integrative Oncology; a full decade before major cancer centers launched integrative medicine clinical programs. It was early innings, and the pushback within academia and across the private practice community within oncology against lifestyle medicine was intense. Suffice it to say, as carefully as I approached the management of my disease, I often felt stranded on a deserted island.

TAKING CONTROL

If I was going to create a comprehensive program to affect the biology of my disease or, at a minimum, supercharge my immune function, I would need to figure it out on my own. And so began my journey to find sensible, evidence-based approaches to improving my overall health and quality of life. In these pre-internet days, books, and articles on the biology of CLL, and early work on the impact of lifestyle changes on disease, were in libraries and bookstores.

Ross Pelton, RPh, CN, became my first 'integrative health' mentor. After reading Ross's *Alternatives in Cancer Therapy*, I went to his home in San Diego for a consultation. He taught me various lifestyle approaches to increase my immune function and to create an environment in my body less hospitable for cancer.

Over time, I would learn about the connection between malignant disease and nutrition, inflammation, oxidative stress, insulin-like growth factor, hydration, metabolism, stress hormones and more.

I became a pescatarian, focusing on a plant rich diet along with cold-water omega-rich fish. My exercise regimen increased: more frequency and a lot more cardio. I installed a whole-house water filtration system, and I arranged for the drinking water supply at my home and office to be outfitted with a reverse osmosis system. I began learning meditation and other forms of stress reduction. Though I had taken various supplements since I was 17 years old, Ross provided guidance around a regimen of supplements and fermented soy to which I closely adhered. I worked with Ross for almost five years, before moving on to another, what I have coined, 'nutritional pharmacologist', a pharmacist who is also a clinical nutritionist.

I met Irwin "Irv" Rosenberg, RPh, CN in late 1999. Irv is the co-founder of what is now called Village Green Apothecary, a single-location sprawling 'compounding pharmacy' located across the street from The National Institutes of Health in Bethesda, Maryland. Irv reviewed my protocol and made several recommendations to fortify my program. Irv invested significant time reviewing the literature for scores of natural products showing anticancer activity. He had relationships with all the major pharma-grade supplement brands and a finger on the pulse of dietary supplement products and development pipeline. It would take a few months to review and understand all the changes Irv recommended and put those into place in early 2000.

BECOMING SICKER

Though my bone marrow had steadily become more involved with leukemic cells, my blood counts were stable, and I felt quite well. I was living a full and active life. That would change in the summer of 2003, a dozen years after my diagnosis. I became ill with Coombs positive hemolytic anemia antibodies that attack red blood cells. My hematocrit dipped to 22.1 My bone marrow was now infiltrated by over ninety percent leukemic cells, crowding out healthy cells.

I made clinic appointments with my local oncologist, Dr. Kressel, MD, and the CLL specialists at Hopkins' Sidney Kimmel Cancer Center in Baltimore. From there I went to Harvard for an appointment with Dr. Nadler at Dana-Farber.

The consensus was clear among my oncology team: I needed to be treated. Immediately. The standard of care had evolved some, and featured the promising new monoclonal-antibody Rituximab, in addition to a couple of chemotherapeutic agents and prednisone.

An autologous bone marrow transplant was no longer offered. Unfortunately, it had not been the curative intervention that people had hoped for. Everyone who had an autologous transplant for CLL would relapse. The experts pushed for therapy to start within a week. Dr. Nadler's words echoed in my head: "Glenn, you are heading over the top of the cliff; you need to be treated now!"

In truth, I felt horrible. I had a constant low-grade fever, was incredibly weak, and woke drenched in a cold sweat three or four times each night. My quality of life was disintegrating. I had a hard time focusing. I needed relief.

EXTENDING THE EXPERIMENT

I told my physicians that I would not submit to conventional therapy. At least not immediately. This decision was based on one simple fact: CLL was still considered incurable. The cocktail of monoclonal-antibody, chemo, and prednisone was essentially a palliative intervention, a Band-Aid until some unknown future treatment. It might put me into a partial remission for a year or two, but the leukemia was certain to return. At that point it would most likely be resistant to the same drug therapy. I was also aware of the potential, lifelong side effects associated with the recommended schema.

I was now a dozen years into my healing experiment. Though I had an underlying severe auto-immune hemolytic anemia (AIHA), and a blood chemistry gone awry, my body was well-conditioned from my extensive integrative oncology regimen.

What are the limits of the body's innate capacity to heal? Could I possibly positively affect my immune function to change the course of this situation?

I told my physicians that while I was not refusing conventional intervention categorically, we would work together over the coming weeks and monitor my blood. If I was unable to impact the course of the AIHA, I would agree to treatment. My oncologists clearly felt I was wasting my time with this approach. However, I had nothing to lose; the standard of care was not curative. But it could deliver relief from my intense suffering. Still, I understood the relationship between my blood chemistry and my feelings well enough to hold off. I trusted that I'd know if and when to nod to that course of treatment.

SABBATICAL AND REVISED REGIMEN

I took a sabbatical from the media company I was running, addressing only the most critical aspects of the business decision-making process. I then revisited my nutraceutical protocol with Irv Rosenberg, eliminating some agents and adding others, such as CLA, artemisinin, and a whey-based immunoglobulin product. Though my anemia was severe, and I was warned about the strain it was having on my heart, I continued with my daily cardio routine of walking and swimming. The activity was short, but happened every day, all outside. It was during these walks and swims that I felt most relaxed. For me, this was the most powerful form of mind/body work. I am simply not the type to sit still and meditate. I tried that early on and struggled to 'turn off the noise'.

ACHIEVING FIRST CLINICAL RESPONSE

Complete blood counts were being done a couple times each week. After several weeks my counts stabilized. After 30 days, there was a clear trend showing improvement. After a couple months, complete blood count (CBC), showed that my blood chemistry had completely normalized. With that news, I had a flow cytometry done locally to take a deeper look at the blood. Flow cytometry analyzes blood to detect the presence of leukemia cells, their type and amount. From a systemic blood flow standpoint there was no evidence of disease.

Some months later, as my full strength returned and I returned to working my previous regular schedule, I went up to Harvard for a PET/CT scan, additional diagnostics, and a physical exam. All confirmed no evidence of disease. I had achieved a partial remission without conventional treatment of any kind. While the systemic blood was clear of leukemia, a bone marrow biopsy revealed my marrow was still impacted by leukemic cells, though greatly reduced since my acute episode.

NOTE: I would later learn that I was the only case in the medical literature showing reversal of AIHA- auto-immune hemolytic anemia, without the aid of steroids or other drug agents.

RELAPSE

I remained in good health and in a partial remission status for six years, until 2009, when the disease recurred.

My white blood cells started increasing; I was anemic, and my absolute lymphocyte count began to rise. From a psychological standpoint it was a challenging period. But I was able to separate the emotional impact from how I was doing physically: asymptomatic and feeling perfectly well. I would approach this news as I had dealt with my illness over many years. I revisited the current standard of care, which had virtually remained static since 2003. I reviewed every aspect of my protocol. I honestly reflected on the current amount of stress in my life.

Earlier, in the summer of 2009, I heard a lecture by Keith I. Block, MD and Penny B. Block, PhD. Thoroughly impressed by the presentation, I read Dr. Block's book, *Life Over Cancer*. Within weeks I was at the Block Center for Integrative Cancer Treatment in Evanston, Illinois (since relocated to Skokie).

At that point I was not 'sick' but had a growing interest in research models. Specifically, I was interested in exploring non-reductive, whole systems, integrative oncology clinical study designs. There was interest at Harvard, and other institutes, to explore a program for CLL, and I felt that bringing in Drs. Keith and Penny Block to collaborate would be a terrific complement for the type of study I envisioned.

Later that year, when I relapsed, I didn't have to give much thought about who I would turn to for help. It was at that point, in the fall of 2009, that I started working with Dr. Block as his patient. He would become my first integrative physician since the onset of my disease 18 years earlier.

RECALIBRATING THE INVESTIGATION

Dr. Block and his team suggested significant changes to my nutraceutical regimen.

Unlike my work with Ross Pelton and Irv Rosenberg, the recommendations Dr. Block made were scientifically informed by my unique biochemical makeup. All the recommendations were based on my macro and micronutrient levels, and various biomarkers connected to hormones, glucose panels, inflammatory load, circulation, and oxidative stress levels.

I adhered to the new supplement protocol for several months, but my white blood count continued to elevate, exceeding 50,000.[2] Ten months into the new protocol, additional changes were made that included clinical dosing of green tea extract (EGCG). We followed the Mayo Clinic dosing of 4 grams daily, which was tolerated well in a phase I study.

ACHIEVING SECOND CLINICAL RESPONSE: COMPLETE REMISSION

After the green tea extract was added, over a relatively short period of time, my white blood counts stabilized. Soon, all areas of my blood chemistry normalized. Flow cytometry showed NED, no evidence of disease in my systemic bloodstream. I had achieved a second clinical response without conventional intervention.

In January 2012, I returned to see Dr. Nadler in the clinic at Dana-Farber. Although not clinically indicated, I insisted on a bone marrow biopsy. From a scientific standpoint it was well-indicated.

I was quite curious to see if my actions had had any measurable impact on the marrow. The pathology came back with the following note:

"Flow cytometric studies of bone marrow and peripheral blood do not reveal diagnostic features of involvement by a lymphoproliferative disorder."

There was no evidence of disease by phenotype or morphology. A Harvard pathologist could not tell that I ever had CLL. In January 2014, I repeated a bone marrow biopsy that showed I was in a complete, durable remission.

I make no claims as to how this complete remission was achieved. I applied a comprehensive, bio-synergistic approach to my disease for over two decades. My outcome does not prove causation. Furthermore, for this article, I have chosen not to share specificity of natural agents, dosing, and how they were informed. It's not been my intention to be prescriptive, but to share my journey purely from a patient's perspective. I do not speculate on pathways, because I do not find it a useful practice. Was it modulation of gene expression, apoptosis, a sustained cytotoxic-like effect from clinical dosing of agents such as EGCG and turmeric? Did the cells simply normalize on their own?

I will never know.

Mine is a story of empowerment and self-efficacy, with a simple message: we are each an n of 1.

Visit GlennSabin.com to download an excerpt from Glenn's book, n of 1, plus receive a bonus guide: 10 Essential Steps to Take Control of Your Cancer Journey.

For more details on Glenn Sabin's clinical case, a peer-reviewed case report was published in December 2015 in Cureus.

https://glennsabin.com/wp-content/uploads/2016/01/Glenn_Sabin_Cureus_case_report.pdf

Glenn Sabin

---

[1] (Hematocrit is a measure of the percentage of red blood cells in the blood. Normal for men is 41% - 50%.)

[2] Normal range is 4,500 – 11,000.

FROM KIDNEY DISEASE TO KIDNEY HEALTH IN 2 MONTHS

SANDRA VANDERMEY

Condition: Kidney disease (stage 3), overweight, sciatica

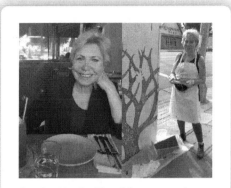

Sandra VanderMey & her artwork

A recognized metalsmith artist, and a teacher of sculpture and metalsmithing at Iowa State University, Sandra VanderMey had her artwork hanging in the Smithsonian and in several Star Trek television programs. Her artwork won many national and international awards. In her late 60's she was diagnosed with stage 3 kidney disease. Everywhere Sandra turned, she was told kidney disease cannot be cured. Available medications could slow its progress but not reverse it. She converted to a whole plant food lifestyle, and in 2 months reversed the disease, to the amazement of the healthcare professionals who said it couldn't be done.

In 1978, when I first began my teaching career I lived with vegetarians and became one myself. It was a much healthier diet than my previous lifestyle of steaks, French fries, smoked links, and burgers, but my doctor said that my vegetarianism was unhealthy! So, I stopped being a vegetarian.

Shortly after this I moved to northwest Iowa to continue teaching, while also pursuing my master's degree. We moved to a town that was 30 minutes away from Sioux City, Iowa, a city with the most slaughterhouses and meat packing plants in the Midwest.

Living where we did at the time, it was difficult not to eat meat! Everyone ate meat. The way I grew up and was used to eating, all meals were centered around meat for breakfast, lunch, and dinner. Meat three times a day. It was a daily staple. When I planned a meal, I started with meat first and then added on the vegetables as a side dish, and in much smaller proportion to the main attraction – meat. If we went out to eat or if we visited friends for dinner, we could not eat a meal where meat wasn't central, particularly red meat. Pork was important as well. Sausage, bacon, pigs in a blanket for breakfast, pork sandwiches for lunch and pork roast for dinner.

We lived next to a hog farm. It often saddened me to look at these innocent creatures and know they were intelligent, sentient beings and that they were grown just so they would one day be slaughtered, and someone could feast on their flesh. Our little town had annual "Appreciation Days," a few days selected in the year when merchants thanked the citizens of the town for their support. Several pigs were killed, put on a spit, and carved up into countless pulled pork sandwiches for the townspeople. I don't think anyone ever thought about the animals they were eating, but I did. Yet like everyone else, I continued to eat meat.

Northwest Iowa had a high rate of cancer, along with other serious diseases, especially amongst younger people. A few people were beginning to link the eating of red meat to their illness. This was particularly true for those with colon cancer, which was probably the most common cancer where we lived.

My child's babysitter, a woman in her early 40's had surgery for colon cancer. To me, she seemed way too young to have any kind of cancer. When she told me her cancer was related to eating too much red meat, it was the first time I had ever heard anything negative about eating meat from an Iowa native. After hearing that, I cut back on eating steaks, hamburgers, and Sunday pot roasts and instead a lot of chicken and fish, which I thought was completely healthy.

At the age of 60, after sixty years of eating meat, I became a long-distance runner thinking that running and limiting my consumption of red meat would help me stay thin and prevent diseases as I got older. But after years of running in competitions, I developed severe sciatica, which eventually landed me in a wheelchair. I began gaining weight because I could no longer exercise. When I had spinal surgery to relieve the pain, it left me semi-sedentary. That created even more weight gain.

I decided I had to do something about my extra pounds, so I visited a nutritionist. She told me the first thing I had to do was get a complete physical exam. It had been a while since my last physical, so after being told this, I was already dreading the results. I was a woman in my late 60s who hadn't had a physical for years. I thought this couldn't result in anything good.

After seeing the nutritionist, I went home that day, and for some reason, my intuition directed me to the Forks Over Knives site. I read everything I could about a whole-food, plant-based diet. This was a seminal moment in my life. I decided at that moment to give it a try. I picked out some recipes from Forks Over Knives, bought groceries and dedicated myself to this new way of living.

I got my physical the day after I started the diet and a week later had the follow-up appointment to review the results of my blood test. That's when my doctor told me the bad news. I had stage 3 kidney disease. When I asked my doctor if there was a cure for kidney disease, she left me with the impression that there wasn't much I could do about it, that it was an inevitable march toward dialysis. She looked skeptically at me when I said maybe my vegan diet could reverse my chronic disease. She referred me to a nephrologist, a kidney specialist.

When I got home, I Googled the definition of "chronic kidney disease" or CKD. I learned that CKD is the slow breakdown of the kidney's ability to filter wastes and fluid from the bloodstream. Everywhere I looked on the Internet, what I read said chronic kidney disease cannot be cured or reversed. Even on the DaVita site, which claims to have the ideal kidney disease diet, it states "chronic kidney disease will not get better." DaVita also said," If you've been diagnosed with CKD, the condition is irreversible."

I could not believe that the go-to site for CKD, gave me only one thing besides meal planning, hopelessness.

Healthline also states, "kidney disease can't be cured" so it wasn't only DaVita that was discouraging.

Talk about despair! I wanted to believe my vegan diet would reverse any damage I had. It seemed my only hope.

The day I saw the nephrologist he was very somber about my previous test results. He said that I had only 44 percent kidney function. That day he did more blood work to follow up on my progress since my last doctor visit. I asked him what I might be able to do to cure the disease, or if I could turn it around. He only said, "We shall see."

What I took him to be saying was: "Don't get your hopes up."

I told him that I had recently switched to a whole food, plant-based diet. He seemed unimpressed but said that it wouldn't hurt.

My test results of CKD consumed me as I continued with my online research. All I could find was that stage 3 kidney disease would steadily progress toward stage 4 kidney disease, and then kidney failure, and dialysis, and maybe a transplant and death. I was three months away from turning 70, and the statistics were even worse for someone my age.

I found a study on several people in my age group with stage 3 three kidney disease. The report said that about half died within three to five years and the rest lived about eight years before they died. I also read that by the time my kidneys failed, I would be considered too old for a transplant. My mom lived to be 92 and I expected to live nearly as long, but unless I could turn this around, I would be lucky if I made it to 78!

Nevertheless, I was still convinced I could at least slow the progression down with my new plant-based diet.

When I looked up what the Internet had to say about a healthy kidney diet, particularly what not to eat if you had CKD, it seemed to conflict with the

DaVita diet. The DaVita diet, which included pre-packaged and canned foods, dairy products, milk, eggs, cream cheese, butter, sour cream, turkey, chicken, fish, red meats, even "kidney friendly candy!" In some cases, DaVita even contradicted itself. I was utterly confused!

I decided it was best to stick to my vegan, whole food, plant-based diet, which seemed to have a built-in, kidney friendly diet.

After all this confusion and discouragement, I fortunately came across a success story from a young woman who completely cured her stage 4 kidney disease with a plant-based diet. I knew then that I, too, could beat the odds.

I continued eating what I thought was the yummiest diet I have ever tried. It was a new way of eating that, regardless of what doctors told me about my health, I would continue forever. I loved the freshness of everything. I could really taste the flavor of the food and found the variety of greens and other salad ingredients tasted better than I had ever experienced. Ever. I never missed meat or dairy products, and I faithfully took vitamin B12 supplements.

Though I was eating well, I still was dreading seeing my nephrologist again, fearful that he would say my new test results indicated my kidney function had dropped even more. I had also gotten an ultrasound and I was scared to see what the results of that might be.

So, at my next appointment, when my nephrologist brought out his laptop, I had real trepidation. He pulled up a chart of my kidney readings over the last twelve years. To my surprise, it showed that most of that time I had been in stage 2 kidney disease, with my kidneys functioning at around 50 percent. No doctor had bothered to mention this to me before! Then he showed me the severe drop on the chart when my kidneys dipped into 44 percent functioning, or stage 3 kidney failure.

But then, with a smile on his face, he showed me the results of my most recent blood tests. My kidneys were functioning at 62 percent!

In the 12 preceding years my kidneys had never functioned that well! He told me that kidneys that were functioning over 60 percent were considered healthy. What's more, he told me, that when he looked at my ultrasound, that it too, displayed completely healthy kidneys.

I said, "I planned on asking you again how to beat stage 3 kidney disease."

His response was, "You already have!"

Though happy for me, the nephrologist was completely puzzled over how this could happen, especially in less than two months!

The biggest surprise for me was when he said, "You're cured. You don't have to see me again."

I told him those good results had to be from me going whole-food, plant based. He told me my diet had nothing to do with it, but I knew in my heart of hearts that it had made all the difference!

After that day, with the passage of time, I went in for more tests and found out my kidneys were now functioning at 67 percent. My most recent blood tests showed my kidneys were functioning at 69 percent! What an amazing transformation, just by going whole food, plant-based! Now I've gone from hopeless to hopeful!

I may never run again, but my physician said I could walk. Nice to know that I now have healthy kidneys.

I've started a walking exercise program and hope to be long-distance running again soon!

Sandra VanderMey

FROM EXTREME RHEUMATOID ARTHRITIS TO EXTREME REVERSAL

CLINT PADDISON

Conditions: Rheumatoid Arthritis, leaky gut

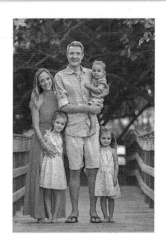

Clint & Melissa
Paddison & Family

Clint Paddison, soon to get married, was diagnosed with aggressive rheumatoid arthritis (RA) at age 31. At first, pain medication helped, but after a year it was no longer effective. He then turned to chemotherapy drugs, which suppress the immune system and its arthritic attacks, but as dosage levels increased, he soon reached the maximum level and still had excruciating pain. When Clint was confronted with the realization that he might never be able to have children, he was motivated to find a solution himself. Accidentally, he discovered that his RA inflammation greatly subsided when he fasted for a day or more. That led him to try different foods to determine which caused inflammation and which did not. He discovered that animal food products and processed, oily foods triggered inflammation, whereas whole plant foods did not. By sticking to a whole plant food lifestyle, Clint reversed his RA such that he came off all medications. Clint and his wife, Melissa, decided to share this healing discovery with others suffering from RA. They created the Paddison Program for Rheumatoid Arthritis which has gone global with over 11,000 users. They have appeared on TV shows, podcasts, TED talks and other forums spreading their message. @ClintPaddison Please visit: **www.paddisonprogram.com**.

One glorious, bright, sunny morning in 2006 I woke up with some strange pain in my feet. The pain persisted, and within a few weeks my fingers began to swell. A local doctor ran my bloodwork which revealed elevated rheumatoid factor, elevated anti-CCP antibodies, and high inflammation markers of CRP and ESR.

"You have rheumatoid arthritis," the doctor said. "RA."

I gave him a blank look. I had never even heard of it. Nobody in my family had this disease, nor anyone I knew. He gave me the lowdown. He said RA is an autoimmune disease where the body's immune system attacks its joints.

He went on to say, "There's no cure and you'll likely be on drugs forever. The goal is to minimize joint damage and try for the best quality of life achievable."

He insisted I see a rheumatologist as soon as possible because "this was serious" and he made a call on the spot to "fast track" an appointment for me in 2 months. I showed up for the rheumatology appointment feeling out of place. There I was, barely 31 years old, in a waiting room with older, debilitated-looking individuals.

The rheumatologist gave me a broad smile and gently shook my hand as if it might be broken. He took a quick look at my blood results and my hot swollen joints and confirmed an RA diagnosis. He then made me acutely aware of the severity of the condition and explained that rheumatoid arthritis is aggressive and progressive. It's nothing like the "wear and tear" osteoarthritis which older people tend to develop. In rheumatoid arthritis, the immune system attacks the delicate tissue surrounding the joints making the joints red, swollen, painful, and tender. This occurs because the lining tissue of the joint becomes inflamed, resulting in the production of excessive joint fluid and thickening of tissue.

Chronic inflammation can cause damage to body tissues, including cartilage and bone. This leads to a cartilage loss and to bone erosion and weakness. That then results in joint deformity, destruction, and loss of function. Ultimately, this can lead to joint replacement if the inflammation remains unmanaged. The doctor explained that since my inflammatory markers were very high, we needed to "address the symptoms aggressively with medications so as to get the disease under control and prevent long term joint damage." He explained that medical management begins with a disease modifying drug, such as methotrexate, a cancer chemotherapy drug, which suppresses the immune system. However, patients often experience increasing dosages or migrate to more powerful drugs in search for one that keeps the disease at bay. Rarely, if ever, do patients reduce their medication. Even rarer still is to get off medication altogether and go "into remission" or be able to go without drugs. The doctor said methotrexate may give me adverse side effects such as fatigue, hair loss, and liver damage (thus requiring monthly blood tests indefinitely). Furthermore, I would not be able start a family due to the drug toxicity.

The doctor asked, "When would you like to start?"

I replied, in total shock. "Can I think about it before starting methotrexate?"

I felt optimistic about being able to improve without methotrexate. I had no family history of rheumatoid arthritis. I had never been seriously sick in any other way. I was the sports captain at my high school and at my university. The rheumatologist accommodated my request to "see how it goes" and reminded me of the severity of my RA. Since I was in a lot of pain, he sent me away with a strong prescription for Diclofenac (an NSAID).

Diclofenac worked amazingly well at eliminating my pain. I remember thinking: "This is IT! All I need to do is take this forever!"

I had no idea, of course, that the effectiveness of the NSAID would wear off. After 3 weeks I was taking more than twice the dosage to get the same pain reduction. I found this very disturbing. So, for my very first RA experiment I decided to see what would happen if I stopped the NSAID's cold turkey.

Oh. My. Gosh! I was in so much agony after skipping the NSAIDs that I was in shock. My pain levels prior to the NSAID had been steadily rising each month, slowly reaching about a 5 out of 10. After three weeks on the NSAID they were now at 8! Horrified by the outcome, I decided right then that I must avoid taking NSAIDs. It was crystal clear to me that they had dramatically worsened my condition. Much later I was to discover that these drugs can indeed worsen the underlying cause of this disease, via exacerbation of a disorder known as "leaky gut." I was afraid of taking methotrexate. I was afraid of taking NSAIDs. I was afraid of high pain levels, and I was afraid I was still getting worse.

I began my search for a natural solution in earnest. I made some basic dietary changes, such as avoiding fast food or occasional unhealthy snacks. I went to see several naturopaths and had live blood analysis, electric currents run through my body to "eliminate microbes at certain frequencies," took countless supplements to eliminate parasitic or bacterial overgrowth and mineral deficiencies, saw Chinese herbalists and acupuncturists, had iridology done on my eyes to determine my inner health, and kinesiology to look for imbalances. I soaked my body in mud baths in Fiji and lay for long periods in thermal hot mineral springs in rural Australia.

During this period, I spent thousands of dollars outsourcing my problem. I did exactly what the experts told me to do. Throughout that year, I woke up every single day believing that I would be better. I was absolutely convinced that the mind has tremendous power over the body, and I was sure that genuine optimism and positive thinking would produce amazing results to turn this condition around.

Yet, at the end of 12 months, I was a disaster. My left knee was so bad I could barely walk. I had inflammation in my chest, so that with every breath I had pain. I had inflammation in my jaw so that with every bite of food I had pain. My fingers and wrists were so sore that I had to use my jaw to pull the covers over me during the night. My elbows were so inflamed and restricted in movement that I struggled to put on my clothes. The elbow pain continued to worsen to the point that when I tried to sleep, I had to suspend my arms with ropes on hooks over my bed.

Reluctantly, I returned to the rheumatologist and conceded that I needed help. He started me immediately on a low dose of Methotrexate (10mg) and suggested we increase the dose as needed. The Methotrexate began to work after 3 weeks, reducing my pain levels by around 70%. However, that remaining 30% was still brutal and over the coming months my situation continued to decline, and my methotrexate dosages continued to rise. The increased dosages were needed to try and control my symptoms and elevated blood inflammation.

Meanwhile, my left elbow had become so heavily inflamed and painful that it became locked into a right-angle position. It was agonizingly painful, like broken glass, if I bumped it or put pressure on it. Consequently, I went in for elbow surgery. The surgery was a significant operation, with two nights in the hospital. This was followed by rehabilitation on a continuous motion machine for 10 hours a day for 6 weeks.

I eventually reached the maximum permissible dose of methotrexate, 25 mg. I was at the doctor's office once more to discuss further drug options. He proceeded to assure me that there were "many more drugs in the cabinet." As the rheumatologist spoke, I realized that the long-term goal of having children was slipping away, and that I was letting my fiancé down. There she sat, beside me once again at the rheumatologist meetings. With my continually worsening condition and poor outlook, I felt like an absolute pathetic failure of a human being and as a life partner. I was ready to explode with suppressed anger and frustration that couldn't be released because my hands, wrists and elbows hurt too much to punch walls.

"F**K THIS S**T!" I kept internalizing. "I can't live like this! I *MUST* get well!"

Right there, in that moment, I decided that I will do everything in my power, anything that my mind could imagine, anything that my body could muster, to get well. There MUST be something I could do to progress out of this living nightmare. I temporarily refused adding more drugs to my therapy, and I returned home driven by fear, anger, and a sense of being backed into a corner, with choices that I refused to accept. I decided to spend my time researching, just like I did at the university, where I studied and researched laser physics. Those years taught me the importance of impeccable scientific methodology in which constants are maintained and only one thing is changed at a time.

I started researching as if I were doing a second university degree. I'd spend hours a day online and ordered books from Amazon as if I were building a library on health and nutrition. My research ramped up with books and medical publications. I bought the only two books I could find on Amazon at the time in which the authors described how they got rid of inflammatory arthritis. I adopted the instructions from both authors exactly as described, but I continued to worsen. Help was scarce, most information online was highly conflicting, and there existed no real path forward for people with this disease.

Fueled by pain, I continued educating myself on gut health, digestive enzymes, stomach acid and anything related to inflammation reduction. I was driven by this whole mystery of "no cause and no cure for RA" spiel from the doctors. It just didn't make sense. I thought, "How could I feel fine for the first 31 years of my life and then feel pain all over in just a few weeks?" Something must have caused it. My physics education taught me Newton's 3rd law: "For every action there is an equal and opposite reaction." Surely then, we are seeing the reaction (joint pains) because of some cause? There MUST be a cause. If I know the cause, I can address it.

Melissa, my wife-to-be, and I continued to obsessively look for answers through research. Melissa has been a vegetarian her whole life, so she encouraged me to shift onto plant-based meals. I noticed an improvement in pain levels. We tested countless supplements, and I introduced a significant amount of exercise since I found that the more, I moved my body the more the pain would subside.

Progress was moderate, but not great, until I got lucky in the strangest of ways. Like many great discoveries, a major breakthrough came by accident. Melissa and I were on a long drive, and we stopped at a supermarket for food. I decided to get some cherries and loaded up on them. I didn't take the time to wash my hands or wash the cherries. I just wanted to get back on the road and eat the cherries. Upon arriving home, I didn't feel too well and had a serious bout of food poisoning. I was violently ill with diarrhea and vomiting for the next 24 hours. During this time in bed, I thought "I'm not moving at all. I'm going to be in such trouble when this passes since my joints will be all stiff and locked up."

However, to my utter shock and delight, when I was done with the purging, I proceeded to get up and walk about with hardly a sore joint to speak of. I was so elated that I literally ran into the city from my house to see my wife and show her my newly re-captured range of motion and pain-free body. This was no small achievement, since at that point I had been unable to run for 3 years!

This experience changed my life. The purging had created such pain relief that it was like a miracle. Yet, when I began eating again the pain came back, and within just a few days it had re-established the same levels in my joints. So, was it specifically the diarrhea or vomiting that helped, or was it just that I had no food inside me? I found out by voluntarily undergoing another fast for 3 days on just celery and cucumber juice. My pain was relieved. This 3-day fast resulted in the same miraculous pain-free outcome, so it confirmed and validated everything that Melissa and I had believed from our studies: The underlying cause of this condition MUST lie in the digestive system. If I don't eat, I feel perfect. If I eat, I feel pain.

My digestion throughout my twenties had not been great. I have had persistent digestive issues ever since I made the unfortunate choice of combating my teenage acne with years of antibiotics. This, I've learned since, is something that shows up quite frequently when reviewing case histories for others with autoimmune diseases. Could it be, we wondered, that everyone with rheumatoid arthritis has serious digestive issues and would get the same pain reduction when fasting? Our research uncovered seven published scientific papers that all showed how fasting dramatically reduced the inflammation of people with rheumatoid arthritis. In some studies, 100% of participants had extremely positive outcomes. We learned that *the symptoms for virtually all RA is strongly linked to the food (or lack of) entering the body.*

This strengthened our belief in the phenomenon of intestinal permeability, or "leaky gut." Undigested food proteins, and bacterial proteins, are entering the bloodstream where they are being identified as an antigen by the immune system, which triggers an immune response and inflammation in the joints. In the absence of these particles in the intestine, and thus the bloodstream, the immune system quickly settles down.

With my recent experience and the science seeming to align, we obsessed over the question: "What can I eat that will give me the lowest possible pain levels?"

The only food that seemed to not add pain and, in fact, reduced pain, was leafy greens. Plain, simple salad greens. So, I decided to eat as many greens as possible in the form of plain salads, and I added sprouts, wheatgrass shots and kept up my cucumber and celery drinks, all which seemed to lower pain.

One thing that stood out to me about these anti-inflammatory foods was that they were raw and uncooked. Extrapolating this, and being motivated by my reading about enzymes, I decided to embark on a completely raw vegan diet for 8 full months. My blood inflammation markers dropped significantly. Since a raw vegan diet was very tough to uphold, after 8 months I was looking for a change. I experimented with quinoa in my diet one evening. Gloriously, I did not experience any pain bump the following day. Encouraged, I was then able to eat quinoa, and shortly thereafter buckwheat, as part of my daily intake.

As the months passed, I was able to maintain my inflammation levels consistently in the normal range. I was aided by daily Bikram yoga, which helped to keep my pain down and restore better functionality to my major joints. Slowly, after many months passed, even the smoldering pain dissipated. I was able to add basmati rice, potatoes, various non-starch vegetables, and eventually beans, legumes, bread, pasta, oats, avocado and virtually every non-processed whole-plant-based food without causing additional pain.

I was able to keep my blood inflammation markers normal for so long that my rheumatologist approved the reduction of methotrexate. As my inflammation markers continued to drop, I was able to get off methotrexate completely. Finally, after being clear of methotrexate for two years, we were able to expand our family. Today, we have three gorgeous, healthy, plant-based children.

I plan to eat an oil-free plant-based diet for the rest of my life. The science suggests that it will lower my risk of heart disease, diabetes, cancer, and other diseases. Over the years, my personal experience and research have shown that it's critical to avoid oils. Just a few years ago I made the mistake to indulge in an oily veggie burger and deep-fried potato wedges at a restaurant. The RA symptoms resurfaced the next morning, and it took me a long time to get my CRP back down to 0.5mg/L. The consequences of this single meal reminded me to never, ever get complacent.

We hope that what I went through to regain my health inspires others.

Clint and Melissa Paddison

FROM FOOD ADDICT TO HEALTH FOOD ADVOCATE

VICTORIA MORAN

Conditions: Obesity, pre-Diabetes, food addiction

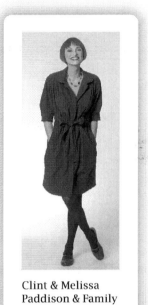

Clint & Melissa
Paddison & Family

Victoria Moran is a vegan of over three decades and was voted "Peta's Sexiest Vegan Over 50" in 2016. Listed by VegNews among the Top 10 Living Vegetarian Authors, Victoria made her reputation in the self-help and spirituality genre with several books, including the international bestseller, Creating a Charmed Life. In the vegan space, she's written many books, including The Love-Powered Diet, The Good Karma Diet, and Main Street Vegan. Featured on Oprah, Victoria is the host of the award-winning Main Street Vegan Podcast. She is the founder and director of the Main Street Vegan Academy, which has trained and certified more than 500 vegan lifestyle coaches, educators, and entrepreneurs since 2012.

Website: *www.mainstreetvegan.net*
Instagram: *@VictoriaMoranAuthor*
Twitter: *@Victoria_Moran*
Main Street Vegan podcast:
On UnityOnlineRadio.org and all major podcast apps

If I set out to find the sixty pounds and pre-diabetic condition I let go of, I'd have to look in the era of Ronald Reagan, *Flashdance, The Big Chill,* and *Terms of Endearment,* a time when it seemed normal to wear leg warmers and shoulder pads and have a perm. Given that the statistical likelihood of keeping weight off for even 5 years is a mere 5 percent, the fact that I'm at thirty-seven years and counting is remarkable.

Moreover, I didn't just have a weight problem: I was a low-bottom binger, eating for a high and dieting as an insidious fix. I first became obese in early childhood, forming all those fat cells that conventional wisdom dictates would doom me to weight issues for life. They have not.

According to family lore, I almost starved in infancy because I couldn't digest milk from a cow or a goat (no one thought of mother's milk in 1950). Buttermilk evidently saved the day. I loved it. Later, I loved most of the foods I was given fried chicken, meatloaf, and hamburgers, cookies, snack cakes, ice cream, scrambled eggs, Wonder Bread and Frosted Flakes (with skim milk, of course, to save on calories).

Calories were a big deal in my house. My father, a physician, had enriched his ear, nose, and throat practice with a thriving "diet doctor" sideline. He tried out all the diets and diet pills on his chubby only child. At one point, he and my mom bought a "reducing salon," featuring the cute "exercise" machines featured in so many ads in the 1950s, with vibrating belts and rotating rollers intended to gyrate the fat away. Of course, it did not involve real exercise. It never worked for me (or anyone else). I was a fat kid and bad for business.

As a teenager, I took over my own weight management. Diet-Rite cola and cottage cheese worked pretty well, until I realized that I could binge on cottage cheese, especially when doused with Sweet 'n Low. My control continued to erode until eventually I could no longer stick with even a "sensible" diet. Other than some marathon water fasts in my twenties, it was easier to eat nothing than to allow a single bite to trigger my addiction. I had just about given up.

I became vegetarian at nineteen, based on a love of animals and an interest in yoga, which recommended a meatless diet. I was able to stay with that, other than one very low afternoon when I devoured a chicken leg from my grandmother's oven. I knew of vegans and wanted to be one, but I slipped and slid in my attempts. It was hard to stand in the 7/11 late at night looking for solace foods, reading labels and finding that everything contained whey or milk powder or egg albumin.

When I tried to pull myself back from a binge, the prevailing sentiment, which cycles through the popular media to this day, was high protein. I ate poached eggs, cheddar cheese and yogurt. I binged on dairy products and then invited back the sugary foods to join in the misery.

At thirty-three, married with a baby daughter, I was desperate for relief. I'd been in and out of Overeaters Anonymous, also known as OA, for almost a decade, but when I went back this time, I surrendered in earnest. The first of OA's 12 Steps says, "We admitted we were powerless over food," and I'd proven that to my own satisfaction. OA would give me principles to overcome addiction. My food plan was to be my choice. Of course, I chose vegan, but this time, because of seriously working the 12 Steps and healing at the desire level, it was possible for me to stay with it, a day at a time, without reaching for food or some other substance.

At that time, "vegan" pretty much meant "whole food, plant based," a term which had not yet been coined. There were a few vegan junk foods; soda, potato chips, Planter's Peanut Bars. Since no one had figured out how to make really good pastries without eggs, being vegan was a great protection against baked goods. No one in the pre-Dr. Ornish 80's was talking about an oil-free diet, but we knew that vegans usually avoided heart disease because we weren't getting cholesterol and saturated fat from animal products.

There were two basic ways that vegans ate back then; either a high-starch, brown-and-beige diet along macrobiotic lines, or a largely raw, Natural Hygiene diet with lots of fruits and vegetables, as popularized by the 1984 mega-seller, Fit for Life. I vacillated between the two and eventually came to a golden mean. Today, I eat whole plant foods selected according to guidance from the time-honored Indian health and healing system of Ayurveda, the sister science of yoga. Grains, starchy vegetables, and easily digestible legumes, red lentils, split mung beans, split pigeon peas, and tofu provided satiety. Vegetables, mostly cooked, plus fruits and berries, some nuts and seeds, and a fragrant array of spices do the rest. The elements are so simple, but the dishes that come from them are glorious.

I adopted OA's advice to eat "three meals a day with living in between" and this continues to serve me well. The problem with food addiction is not so much starting to eat as stopping once you've started. Sticking with breakfast, lunch, and dinner is not a religious edict for me, and if a meal is delayed, I'll eat a piece of fruit with a few nuts, or drink a green juice.

I realize this is not a "whole" food, but green juice with lemon makes me feel as if I'm sipping from the fountain of youth, and I do so most days.

I refrain from alcohol. I figure if I could develop an addiction to food, I'm not someone to cozy up to booze. I keep processed foods to the bare minimum, allowing them in as a travel compromise. I'm on the road a lot for my work. I'm vegan away from home, of course, but bread, veggie-burgers, power bars, and sometimes white rice are on the out-of-town menu. I make a point to accept and enjoy whatever I eat. I spent thirty-three years in guilt and remorse, and I've now lived even longer without it.

At seventy-one, I take no pharmaceuticals and I've avoided the health problems that plagued members of my family long before they reached this age.

I realize that health is about more than food and I can't predict the future, but "just for today," to borrow some 12 Step vernacular, I am healthy and grateful.

Victoria Moran

FROM DEADLY DIABETES TO NEW LIFE
MARC RAMIREZ

Conditions: Diabetes, Obesity, high cholesterol, hypertension, psoriasis, erectile dysfunction, sleep apnea, GERD

With almost his entire family devastated by diabetes, heart disease, obesity, high blood pressure, and other diseases, Marc Ramirez figured he was destined for the same fate. Everyone believed that Hispanic genes would cause him to suffer the same diseases. When he was diagnosed with diabetes, he was told he would be on medications for the rest of his life. His mother and every one of his siblings died or had horrendous consequences from diabetes and other diseases. Fortunately for Marc, his in-laws gave him a copy of the iconic Forks Over Knives documentary. That led him to read Dr. Neal Barnard's Program for Reversing Diabetes. Marc and his wife, Kim, converted to a whole food, plant-based lifestyle. Within 2 months, Marc was off all diabetes medications. Marc and Kim now share their story with others who are still suffering. They founded a non-profit called Chickpea and Bean to promote their healing message through free meetings, seminars, online Plant Plunges, and nutrition and cooking classes. Please visit: **www.ChickpeaAndBean.com**.

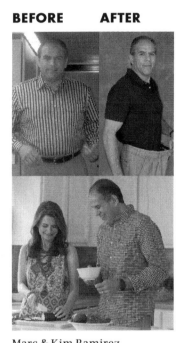

BEFORE   AFTER

Marc & Kim Ramirez

"You will be on insulin the rest of your life."

"You're Hispanic, diabetes is in your genes, and you can't do anything about it."

Or so I was told.

And why not believe these statements? As a child I remember members of my family battling diabetes, heart disease, cancer, high blood pressure, and high cholesterol. Sometimes dying from these diseases or losing their limbs or eyesight to them. And always suffering from them.

I grew up at the tip of southern Texas with four brothers and three sisters. When I was eight years old, my father abandoned our family and my mother struggled to raise eight children on her own. In search of better employment, she decided to move us to the Chicago area in 1982.

In high school I thrived as an athlete and earned a football scholarship to the University of Michigan. Because I was so physically active back then, I could eat whatever I wanted and did not have health issues. At twenty-one years old I was 6'2" and weighed 305 pounds.

While I played for Michigan and pursued my degree, my mother battled diabetes and her health gradually declined. She suffered from vision problems, high cholesterol, high blood pressure, heart disease, and kidney failure. In 1995 she underwent kidney transplant surgery. Jill is our only sibling who never developed diabetes, but she, too, felt its impact as she bravely donated a kidney to our mother.

Diabetes also caused my mother's heart disease to worsen and years later she needed a double bypass. She had the surgery and passed away a few days later. After over 33 years of fighting diabetes, my mother passed away in April 2002. She was the family rock, and I miss her dearly.

Everyone in my family struggled with deadly chronic diseases. If that were not bad enough, my oldest brother David passed away in June 2002, just 2 months after my mother, due to pancreatic cancer. My twin brother, Joe, battled diabetes for over 16 years and had a heart attack. Sandra, my youngest sister, also has type 2 diabetes. Martin, our youngest sibling, suffers greatly from diabetes. He had pancreas and kidney transplants, is legally blind, had his right leg amputated, goes to dialysis three times a week. He takes 25 medications every day. My oldest sister, Carol, though, who also struggled with diabetes, started eating mostly plant-based foods and eliminated her medications.

As the years progressed, I put on pounds and found myself having high hemoglobin A1c C levels. The hemoglobin A1c test is familiar to people with diabetes. It measures the average glucose levels in the blood over a 2-to-3-month period. It indicates how much glucose remains in the blood and ultimately determines if medications are needed. Doctors consider someone diabetic and if they need to start medications based primarily on their A1c level. The current A1c range for a non-diabetic is between 4.0 and 5.6. If the A1c level is between 5.7 – 6.9, the person is considered pre-diabetic. An A1c level of 7.0 or higher is considered full blown diabetes.

I began taking the diabetes medication, Metformin, in 2002. My A1c level back in 2002 was 8.8 and ultimately rose to as high as 10.5 in September 2011. I was on insulin injections (Lantus) and I had already been taking four oral medications for years, Metformin (for diabetes), Januvia (for diabetes), Simvastatin (for high cholesterol), and Lisinopril (for high blood pressure). During my decade of being sick and obese, I also developed ED (erectile dysfunction), psoriasis, frequent heartburn, and possibly sleep apnea because I did not sleep well.

As my A1c levels gradually rose over the years, I tried to improve my health by dieting, exercising more, and cutting carbs. Unfortunately, these strategies did not stop the progression of diabetes. (Later I learned that carbs are not my enemy—fat is.) Eventually, my doctor told me that I had to begin injecting insulin daily.

I found myself feeling frustrated and helpless. For years I had witnessed my family suffering from diabetes. I saw myself as destined to walk down the same path. I believed there was no cure, and that diabetes was just something the members of my family had to deal with. And die from.

I remember asking my doctor if I would ever stop taking the insulin injections and his response was, "No, you will be on insulin for the rest of your life."

This really pissed me off. I felt helpless. It seemed as though diabetes was inevitable because I'm Hispanic and belong to a culture with a high rate of diabetes, and my family was filled with diabetics. So, I reluctantly accepted the fact that I was fated to have the same disease because of my genetic heritage.

In the autumn of 2011, my in-laws gave my wife, Kim, and I a copy of the DVD, *Forks Over Knives*. One day, feeling somewhat hopeless and defeated about my health problems, Kim and I decided to watch it. This inspirational documentary gave us hope and persuaded us to try a whole food, plant-based way of life. I also purchased the book *Dr. Neal Barnard's Program for Reversing Diabetes*.

On December 3, 2011, we both went vegan. My life and health changed dramatically. I now follow three basic guidelines for eating: (1) I eat no animal products, (2) I eat low-fat foods, and (3) I avoid high glycemic foods.

I enjoy foods such as oatmeal with cinnamon and raisins, pasta primavera with marinara sauce, bean burritos with jalapeno peppers, veggie subs, black bean burgers, and plenty of fruits and vegetables such as strawberries and sweet potatoes. Notice that this is not a low carb diet. I enjoy a lot of complex carbs. Carbs are not the enemy. High fat foods are. Fat gets in the muscle cells and prevents insulin and glucose from working properly.

In less than two months after adopting a whole food plant-based lifestyle, I was off all my medications. I've remained medication-free for years now. All my conditions mentioned earlier have disappeared and the weight has not returned. When I began this journey, I weighed 254 pounds and today I weigh 207 pounds, which was what I weighed in seventh grade. I am grateful to say that I am no longer diabetic. And eating plant-based has kept me hard below the waist.

I now know that it is not because I am Mexican or because my family is genetically predisposed to diabetes that I suffered from this disease. It all comes down to the daily choices I make of how to nourish my body with the food I eat. By cutting out the foods that are nutrient poor and replacing them with foods that are nutrient rich, my body responds positively.

My wife and I are empowered and liberated by our new lifestyle. We feel strong, healthy, and in charge of our lives. This lifestyle improves our health, helps prevent cruelty to animals, combats hunger issues, and is better for the environment.

While Kim and I feel thrilled with our results, we also feel frustrated. Why did no health care provider ever suggest plant-based nutrition? Why is this way of eating met with such criticism and skepticism? Why don't doctors know this?

Why did I have to get this message from a documentary instead of a doctor?

After all, the Hippocratic Oath states, "I will apply dietetic measures for the benefit of the sick." Hippocrates said, "Let food be thy medicine." Why aren't doctors following these dictums?

Kim and I strive to spread the message and let others know that going plant-based might help them, too. We began a nonprofit called Chickpea and Bean. Our mission is to educate people about the benefits of a plant-based lifestyle.

For more information, please go to www.ChickpeaandBean.com

We would love to help you too.

Marc Ramirez

FROM MR. BBQ TO PLANT-BASED NUTRITION THERAPIST

BRIAN DEVON

Conditions: Chronic kidney disease, heart disease, atrial fibrillation, arrhythmia, hypertension, overweight

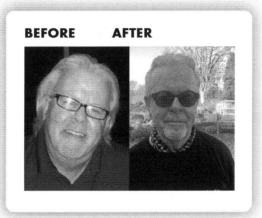

BEFORE   AFTER

Brian Devon had been a cook who emphasized meat and animal-based foods. But then he had a series of health events: atrial fibrillation, arrhythmia, and hypertension. The whopper was a diagnosis of moderate kidney disease, which according to his doctor was not reversible. Brian went on a keto diet – low carb, high protein diet – the kind of diet he thought he would love because it had lots of his favorite food, meat. But very quickly he found himself not feeling well, and when he had blood work done, he was shocked to learn that his kidney disease had rapidly deteriorated from moderate to severe. By chance he came upon the iconic documentary, Forks Over Knives. *He watched it and realized it held the answer to his problems. He converted to a whole food, plant-based lifestyle and within months his bloodwork demonstrated results that, according to his physicians, were not possible. His severe kidney disease had improved to a "mild" level!*

The first warning that things were not right with my health was when I felt my heart **STOP!**

It was my first cardiac arrhythmia. I was sitting at the computer desk mid-morning. Suddenly, my heart just stopped. That's what it felt like. It stopped and then it started. A second later it started with a thud, and then it was racing at 180 beats-per-minute.

This was atrial fibrillation, a form of cardiac arrhythmia, a condition that affects 6 million Americans. Atrial fibrillation is commonly referred to as "afib" and the Standard American Diet, the "SAD" diet, can be one of the causes. The SAD diet is high in animal food products that lead to cardiovascular disease, cancer, autoimmune diseases, and countless other ailments. It is killing us all.

When I tried to stand up from my computer desk while suffering from atrial fibrillation, I fell over. I was very dizzy and unstable. I called my doctor's office immediately and they said to come in right away. On arrival there, they checked me out and sent me to the Emergency Room at a nearby hospital.

For many years before, I had been "Mr. BBQ." I never missed an opportunity to get the grill fired up! I was a bacon-and-eggs type of guy at breakfast. Obviously, I loved meat. I even went on a Paleo "caveman" diet for a time to further enjoy my bounty of meat.

Then, during a routine blood work-up, I was told my kidney function was not good. This, combined with my atrial fibrillation, was really worrying me. I was already on four blood pressure medications, and my weight had crept up to where I was 30 pounds overweight. So, having kidney problems on top of all this was not good news. The doctor told me: "This is serious, but not yet an emergency."

I was referred to a nephrologist, a kidney specialist, who told me after more blood work, that my eGFR was 42, which was not good. I had chronic kidney disease at a moderate level. I'll explain. GFR stands for glomerular filtration rate. It is a key measure of kidney function. GFR tests are hard to do, so most labs provide an eGFR number from blood tests. That is an estimated GFR based on a patient's creatinine level, age, sex, and race. The desirable normal level is 90 or above for younger people, lowering to 60 or above for older people. A reading below 60 indicates kidney disease. With an eGFR of 42, I was at a moderately diseased level. This, along with my other problems, was not good.

The kidney doctor said my disease was irreversible and the best I could hope for was to slow the decline. Kidney disease is a progressive disease; it gets worse over time. Drugs cannot cure it, only slow down the progression, at best.

Over the next year my atrial fibrillation became more frequent and more persistent. I was becoming a poster boy for the western SAD diet.

I went to a cardiologist who tried meds to treat the atrial fibrillation. He gave me Flecainide, to which I reacted badly. Flecainide is a drug that is supposed to stop or reduce atrial fibrillation, but it caused my blood pressure to shoot up to 197/110. I was concerned, to say the least. I had a family history of strokes. Both my sister and my father had died from strokes at age 58.

After being discharged from the hospital for the arrhythmia, I was taking Diltiazem 180 mg twice daily for high blood pressure, Nebivolol 5 mg once daily, also for high blood pressure, Losartan 100mg once daily, yet again for high blood pressure, and Bendroflumethiazide 2.5 mg, a diuretic for the kidneys and for the high blood pressure. Also, Xarelto 15mg once daily, a blood thinner administered to prevent blood clots from forming. Did I mention I had high blood pressure?

I was told that in addition to the high blood pressure, I had serious kidney problems because my Albumin/Creatinine ratio was 155.8; eGFR was 42; CRP was 33.5 mg/L; and my triglycerides were 662. The triglycerides on a previous test had been a ridiculously high of above 1200.

To put all this into proper perspective, understand that Albumin/Creatinine ratio, which is another measure of kidney function, is considered normal if it is under 30. Mine was over 155. Normal eGFR is over 90 for younger people, and over 60 for older folks. Mine was 42. Normal CRP, or C-Reactive Protein, is under 1. Mine was an extraordinarily high 33.5 mg/L. CRP is a measure of inflammation levels in the body. The higher it is, the worse condition the body is in, and a heart attack or stroke could be imminent. Normal triglycerides, which are a measure of certain fats in the bloodstream, are less than 150. Mine were off the charts at 662. I was a real mess!

I suppose I could be called a foodie, or a meaty foodie. So, my first inclination was to look at dieting. I took a hard look at the Keto diet, which I thought would suit me perfectly because I wouldn't have to give up meat, my favorite food. So, I started a strict Keto diet and within a couple of weeks I had lost about 5 lbs. But I was not feeling very good.

I decided to get blood work done to check up on my kidney function. I was horrified to find that I had deteriorated to an eGFR of 33. I had gone from moderate kidney disease to severe kidney disease on a Keto diet! I was told if my eGFR fell below 30, I should discuss dialysis and kidney transplant options with the nephrologist. This came as a real shock!

At the same time as all this was happening, I got a notice from Netflix that the documentary film, *Forks Over Knives*, was about to be removed from Netflix, so I thought I'd watch it. What a revelation! Here was the solution to metabolic problems right in front of me! I then bought the book, *The China Study*, by T. Colin Campbell, Ph.D., on which much of the information in *Forks Over Knives* was based. Overnight, I literally became a whole food, plant-based eater. For the next 12 weeks I followed *Forks Over Knives'* whole plant food diet religiously.

I recently got my first bloodwork results based on this lifestyle.

The results are amazing. My eGFR went up from 33 to 50! I went from severe kidney disease to moderate disease, and not far from mild kidney disease. My uric acid is normal. Creatinine is normal. Triglycerides are now normal at less than 150 mg/dL, after they were a terrible 1200 mg/dl.

According to my doctors this cannot happen, not with medications or any other way. But it did.

When I called for the test results, I spoke to the practice manager at the doctor's office who started reading the results, and then stopped and said, "This is amazing!"

(They knew I was on the whole plant food diet and approved of it wholeheartedly. The doctor's son is vegan).

The practice manager said, "I want to show this to the doctor."

A few minutes later the doctor called and said, "This is unbelievable! I have never seen such dramatic results."

To cap it all, I've lost 34 pounds and have gone from 4 blood pressure meds to 2. I've even cut the dosages of those 2 blood pressure meds. (90 mg Diltiazem and 100mg Losartan are my only blood pressure meds now.) My average blood pressure now is 112/70. I haven't had any atrial fibrillation since I started the whole plant food diet. This is truly a miracle!

I've been eating whole plant foods morning, noon, and night. Quite a switch from my meat-eating days. I've gone from eggs and bacon for breakfast to oats and fresh fruits. I eat a lot of apples and pears every day. No more meat or BBQ at lunch or dinner, either. Now, I have whole grains such as quinoa and buckwheat, or vegetables such as cauliflower, green beans, broccoli, zucchini, and carrots. My wife and I also enjoy making homemade flatbreads and eating them with hummus, tomato, and bell peppers.

My daughter was so impressed with how rapidly I lost weight and improved my health that she became a whole plant food lifestyle person as well.

I had been cooking up a storm at home and for friends for years in my meat-eating days. People knew that to buy me a cookbook as a gift was a surefire winner, and it was common for them to suggest, "You should open a restaurant." So, I did.

My wife, Jane, and I opened our own restaurant in a tourist destination. It was a little gem and quite a success, in season. Unfortunately, winters were quite a challenge, so after two successful summer seasons we said goodbye to the restaurant and focused on catering and other cooking gigs.

In those days, meat was a focal point. Back then, protein was the core of what every commercial chef produces, and the most popular source of protein was meat. But when I was awakened to plant-based healthy living, I decided to embark on a journey to become a Nutritional Therapist.

I pursued a course in Clinical Nutrition to understand how a whole plant food diet works to produce better health. I wanted to know how to continue using nutrition as I got older, to maintain my good health. Finally, I wanted to help people I met, or who heard about me, improve their health, and manage their weight through a whole plant food lifestyle. I've gone from being Mr. BBQ to being a plant based Nutritional Therapist. I couldn't be happier.

As I said, this transformation has been a miracle for me. It can be a miracle for anyone. There is nothing special about me. It is all about a whole food, plant-based diet.

Doctors will tell you that kidney disease is irreversible. That's what my doctor told me. Don't believe it for a second. Most doctors don't know anything about healthy, plant-based nutrition. Nutrition is not studied in medical schools.

Kidney disease can be reversed. High blood pressure can be reversed. Cardiovascular disease can be reversed. Chronic diseases can be reversed.

A whole food, plant-based diet will do all of that. For everyone.

Spread the word.

Brian Devon

AVOIDING STENTS AND CARDIAC BYPASS SURGERY

JIMMY CONWAY, M.D.

Conditions: Heart disease, high cholesterol, high triglycerides, hypertension

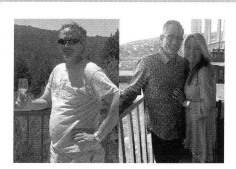

Dr. Jimmy Conway, an orthopedic surgeon, was facing the prospect of triple bypass cardiac surgery because an arteriogram image had revealed blockages in his coronary arteries that were too large to stent. He had just read The China Study, by T. Colin Campbell, Ph.D., one of the leading nutrition scientists in the country. Dr. Conway was angry that he had never been taught that animal-based foods promote disease and that plant-based foods prevent

Dr. Jimmy Conway – before & after with wife, Andrea

disease, even though this information has been known for decades. Dr. Conway rejected having bypass surgery and instead converted to a whole food, plant-based diet. In six months, he reversed his heart disease, passed the stress test he had previously failed, and his cholesterol fell by almost 80%. He began teaching patients about a plant-based lifestyle to reverse and prevent disease. He and his wife, Andrea, launched **www.plantbasedokc.com**. *Dr. Conway recently became certified by the American College of Lifestyle Medicine. After retiring from orthopedic practice, he hopes to devote full time to lifestyle medicine, where he feels that he is really healing people.*

My name is Jimmy Conway, and I am an orthopedic surgeon. An orthopedic surgeon with a strong family history of heart disease.

My father had multiple stents, a bypass surgery and more stents starting at the age of 50. When he finally passed away, he was on dialysis three times a week, in constant pain and had an ejection fraction of less than 10%.[1]

I had countless other male and female relatives that died of heart attacks or strokes. With that history, when I awoke with left arm pain one morning, I knew that was not good. I was on three different anti-hypertensives (blood pressure medications) that, as a physician, I was managing myself.

Surprisingly, I had never had my cholesterol or other lab work drawn. Physicians look after the health of other people, but they are notorious for ignoring their own health. After the left arm pain episode, I made an appointment with a cardiologist. The first thing he did was draw blood and send it to the lab for analysis. My total cholesterol came back as 494, and my triglycerides were over 3,200!

My cardiologist said he had never seen triglycerides that high. The guidelines for "normal" cholesterol and triglycerides are less than 200 and 150, respectively. That meant that my cholesterol was 2 ½ times normal and my triglycerides were more than 21 times normal!

I was then scheduled for a treadmill stress test which I failed. That meant I had adverse EKG changes while on the treadmill before I could even get my heart rate up. The next step was to do an arteriogram, sometimes called an angiogram. This is a procedure in which a catheter is inserted through an artery from the groin or the wrist and snaked up to the heart. A contrast dye is pumped through the catheter into the coronary arteries surrounding the heart. The contrast dye makes the coronary blood flow highly visible on X-Ray monitors placed above the heart. The cardiologist can easily detect blockages in the coronary artery, how severe they are and where they are located.

Looking back, I think how naïve I was. Several of my physician partners were in their 50's and they had had cardiovascular events resulting in stents. This was what I considered "normal," right?

On the Friday afternoon before the Monday on which the arteriogram was scheduled, my wife met one of my partners. She mentioned to him I would be having this test on Monday. He told her to get the book, *The China Study*, by Dr. T. Colin Campbell. She got the book that night from the local bookstore. I spent the entire next day, Saturday, immersed in this book.

The China Study clearly and eloquently describes how an animal-based, processed food diet is behind the myriad chronic diseases that afflict billions of people worldwide. Especially cardiovascular disease and cancer. Dr. Campbell presents abundant scientific data to demonstrate how animal-based diets promote disease, and how plant-based diets prevent and even reverse disease. The more I read the angrier I became. This information had been known for decades! Yet as a physician, and having gone through medical school for four years, and more years as an intern, I had NEVER heard anything like it. Why?

Monday morning came and we went to the heart hospital and checked in for the arteriogram. My wife and I both thought they would more than likely place a few stents, we would go home, tweak our diet and life would go on. No big deal.

Instead, I woke up from the procedure with the cardiothoracic surgeon looking over me. Not a good sign. The cardiologist stated I had a 70% blockage of my right main coronary, an 85% blockage in my left anterior descending artery, which is known as the Widowmaker, and an 80% blockage further downstream. It is known as the Widowmaker because it is the main culprit in fatal heart attacks. According to my cardiologist these blockages were too large to stent, and he was recommending triple bypass surgery, the sooner the better.

My wife and I were in shock. This was not on our radar. I was scheduled for surgery that Friday, four days later. On the way home, I told my wife there is a book mentioned in the China Study called *Prevent and Reverse Heart Disease* by Dr. Caldwell Esselstyn of the Cleveland Clinic. I wanted to read that book!

I was off work the next day, due to the arteriogram procedure, so we got the book and I read it. Again, I was blown away by the information. Who knew you could reverse heart disease? Never had I heard of the concept of reversing heart disease from any physician, let alone a cardiologist.

I knew I did not want to end up like my dad or worse, so my wife and I decided right there and then that surgery was out of the question. We were going all in. 100% whole food, plant-based.

The next day, at the follow up appointment with the cardiologist, I told him of our decision. The cardiologist was not happy. He reluctantly agreed after giving me liquid nitroglycerin in case of an emergency.

So, in October of 2009 our journey into a whole food plant-based lifestyle began and we haven't looked back. After 6 months eating a whole food, plant-based diet with no added oil, my cholesterol dropped to 115, my LDL was 15 which is the lowest the test can measure, and my triglycerides went to 175. I also did a repeat stress test, which I passed. After about 2 years I weaned off all hypertensives and statins. My last bloodwork showed both my cholesterol and triglycerides to be under 100 each.

Now, as a more enlightened physician, and in my own personal practice as an orthopedic surgeon, I know that most of the problems I treat are the result of the "Standard American Diet." I believe a rotator cuff tear to be a "heart attack" of the shoulder. The exact mechanisms that cause heart attacks are the same ones that cause the rotator cuff to tear.

Healthy blood vessels mean a healthy life!

Jimmy Conway, M.D.

---

[1] Ejection fraction is a measure of the heart's pumping efficiency, roughly equal to the amount of blood pumped out on each beat as a percentage of the amount coming into the heart. An ejection fraction of 50% or higher is considered normal. An ejection fraction of 10% or less, like my father had, is near-term fatal.

FROM FAST FOOD ADDICTION TO FREEDOM

EMILY BOLLER

Conditions: Obesity, food addiction, anorexia, heart disease, hypertension, pre-diabetes, trauma, grief, bereavement, PTSD

Emily Boller was desperate to find freedom from her struggles with food. She had experienced chubbiness in childhood, anorexia in her teens, and obesity in her adult years. Then she read Eat to Live, the bestselling book by Dr. Joel Fuhrman, and began documenting her 100-pound weight loss journey. At that time, she never expected to become a voice of inspiration for food addiction recovery. Today, she considers herself to be a guide for anyone who wants to scale the mountain of food addiction and poor health. Emily combines her personal journey, hard-won wisdom, and practical tips with nutritional science to help others break free from the misinformation that sabotages health and well-being. After losing a child to suicide, she knows how trauma, grief, crisis, and stress impact recovery from addiction and how to recover from relapses as well. Please visit: **www.EmilyBoller.com** *or contact* **Emily@EmilyBoller.com**.

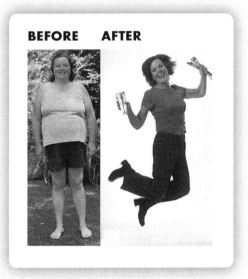

BEFORE   AFTER

"Change only happens when the pain of not changing is greater than the pain of changing."

I had struggled with an addiction to food since early childhood. I was chubby as a kid, which changed to anorexia in my late teens and then back to obesity in my adult years.

By age 42, I was obese and experiencing chest pains and shortness of breath. I had a heart catheterization and was officially diagnosed with coronary artery disease. And I still had five children at home to raise. I wanted to get healthy. I had already tried every diet imaginable, and nothing worked long-term. In fact, I always gained more weight back afterward, so I just quit trying to lose weight altogether. Not realizing this at the time, I had been struggling with food addiction as the root of my weight problems my entire life.

Five years later, I was more than 100 pounds overweight. By now, I had developed pre-diabetes on top of the heart disease. I was lethargic and increasingly immobile.

My midsection had become so bloated and large that I couldn't roll over easily in bed, or fit into a pop-up tent, or squeeze into the backseat of a 2-door sedan. I even broke and fell through a nylon folding chair at one of my kid's soccer games! I was beginning to feel like a bull in a china closet.

In March 2018, just before my 47th birthday, while waiting for a prescription to be filled at Walmart, I put my arm into one of those blood pressure machines that are in many pharmacy waiting areas. The machine registered my blood pressure as 154/94. Seeing those numbers was my wake-up call. *I knew I had to change.* Both of my parents had heart attacks, my dad had heart bypass surgery, and my mother and maternal grandmother had debilitating strokes.

I knew I was sitting on a ticking time bomb — not a matter of "if" I would have a heart attack or stroke, but "when." My youngest child was only ten. I knew I had to make a change ASAP. But even with that motivation, the addiction to food was stronger than my desire to change. I was stuck in a hole, digging my grave instead.

Then, two days before my 47th birthday, I visited my friend Audrey's studio. We are both artists. She and I had met two years before on a university-sponsored trip to study the art of Italy and Greece from the Renaissance period. On that trip I got to see the many masterpieces I had studied in Art History years ago. When I stepped into the vault of the Sistine Chapel and looked up, I couldn't move. I had studied the paintings in books but was totally unprepared for the emotional experience of viewing it in person. No one speaks in that chapel. No one wants to speak. No one is allowed to speak. The silence protects vibrations from damaging the images.

From that moment onward, I felt very conflicted as an artist. I wouldn't think of smearing mud on Michelangelo's masterpieces. But here I was, smearing mud daily on the greatest masterpiece of all -- my own body. I was desecrating my body daily with the destructive food I was choosing to put into it. Back in Audrey's studio, I had an idea: *What would happen if I used food as an artistic medium? Just as a painter uses paint, or a sculptor uses stone, or a potter uses clay . . . I would use food to fashion my body into the work of art that it was originally meant to be.*

The idea seemed to me like divine inspiration. It was a catalytic moment that lit a flame deep within me, and the clarity of that vision was unstoppable. Right there, in her studio, an art exhibit was born. An exhibit that would use food as the artistic medium and my obese body as the point of departure. I would name it *Transformation.*

I read Eat to Live by Joel Fuhrman, M.D. and knew instantly that I would follow the nutritional information in that book as my impetus for change. Dr. Fuhrman teaches that when the body is properly nourished, cravings for unhealthy foods dissipate, and then eventually go away. I knew that if I got rid of the cravings for the foods that were destroying my body, I'd be able to reclaim my health.

I began the art exhibit of my body on the morning of July 10, 2008, with a visit to my family physician. He ordered a blood test for me to have a baseline for my personal art exhibit. I documented my month-to-month progress online, including medical stats and images of my changing body size. I announced the art exhibit to everyone; friends and strangers alike were following it. Within a year, I had lost 100 pounds, but more importantly, I had gotten rid of the food addiction that had been holding me back from living life to the fullest. I also eradicated coronary artery disease and pre-diabetes.

I became athletic. I jogged six miles most days, I bought a bike and rode for pleasure, I hiked rugged trails with my teens and even ran my first 5K race. For the first time in my life, I was free from food addiction! Eventually, the art exhibit went viral and inspired individuals from all over the world. In the year that I was losing weight, I joined Dr. Fuhrman's member center, which is an online support community of individuals following *Eat to Live*. This included the ability for members to ask Dr. Fuhrman questions and interact with him.

At the one-year milestone, Dr. Fuhrman asked if I could write 500 words about my favorite vegetable. He wanted to post it on his blog. So, I wrote about romaine lettuce. His readers enjoyed it, so he asked if I could write another one related to my weight-loss journey. So, I did . . . and again, his readers enjoyed it. This continued for three more months. What started out as a simple posting on Dr. Fuhrman's blog snowballed into a weekly post for the next *four years!* My writings reached thousands of readers.

Then, Dr. Fuhrman invited me to speak at his health retreats, as well as on TV, including *The Dr. Oz Show.* Ten days after the taping of *The Dr. Oz Show,* my 21-year-old son died by suicide on Memorial Day 2012. The show aired to millions of viewers two days before the funeral.

After the initial shock wore off, I experienced symptoms of PTSD: fitful nights of sleep, uncontrollable crying spells, intestinal disturbances, fear of things I had never been afraid of before. By mid-August, I was somewhat able to travel and speak again. I wanted to prove my resilience, so I continued to write weekly blog posts, speak in churches, and travel . . . until I hit a wall eighteen months later. I couldn't function. My world turned dark. I was exhausted and my legs felt like bags of sand. I couldn't even brush my teeth on some days. I lost all desire to carry on. Apathy set in and I didn't even care about my health anymore. I gained some weight back. I didn't care about that or anything most days. But then, with each additional pound gained, my anxiety skyrocketed. I felt ashamed of my lack of self-control; not realizing I was running away from processing the trauma and grief.

Four days before Christmas 2016, I experienced some fluttering in my chest, so I took my blood pressure. It had skyrocketed to dangerous levels of hypertension. I laid down on my bed and didn't move . . . for the next five days, including Christmas Day. I drank only water, hoping to bring my blood pressure down to safe levels. The day after Christmas my blood pressure was still dangerously high, so I asked my husband to drive me to the ER. I was so afraid that I couldn't even speak to the security officer at the door. He asked if I needed assistance, and I could only answer him with motions.

The ER staff immediately hooked me up to check my vitals. I knew for sure that I'd be having bypass surgery that day. In that ER cubicle, I regretted every careless meal I had eaten after my son died. I knew I was paying the price for those mistakes. But after a 3-hour wait, a doctor slid the curtain aside and told me I could go home. There was nothing wrong with my heart. I had experienced a panic attack.

What?!!! A panic attack?!!!

Instantly, I wanted to do cartwheels all the way out the door! I wanted to live again . . . and live well!

Since then, I have added more tools to my recovery from food addiction. Eating the correct food again was important, but I also added support groups, grief counseling, prayer support, meditation, and massage. I made a good night of sleep a top priority. The "bereavement fat" I had gained is slowly coming off. The complicated weight of grief is lifting, and I am now genuinely happy to be alive again.

Now, I can encourage anyone who is suffering from trauma or profound loss of any kind: *There is hope.* With proper care, broken, traumatized hearts can heal.

For anyone who has suffered years with debilitating struggles with food addiction and/or eating disorders, recovery is possible, but it takes vigilant intent to adhere to the recovery lifestyle. There will be setbacks and lapses in judgement at times for most people, and that's normal. The key to lifelong freedom is to quickly wipe away the mistakes and keep going.

Never give up!

Emily Boller

FROM DOCTOR TO PLANT-BASED NUTRITIONIST
LEILA DEHGHAN-ZAKLAKI, M.D.

Conditions: Migraines, headaches, overweight, bulimia, analgesia addiction and withdrawal, gastritis, constipation

Dr. Leila Dehghan-Zaklaki suffered from horrendous migraine headaches from an early age. She suffered an ordeal of many years, where she tried every imaginable solution to the debilitating headaches that sidelined her for half a month or more, every month. This ordeal finally came to an end when she discovered the healing powers of whole plant foods. Today, she is a doctor turned plant-based nutritionist. She received her medical degree from the University of Vienna and completed her internship in the UK. Her personal experiences of overcoming health challenges through diet shifted her professional interests to focus on the power of nutrition. She earned a Plant-Based Nutrition Certificate at e-Cornell and obtained a M.S. degree in Clinical and Public Health Nutrition from the University College of London. She takes a holistic approach to her clients' needs and helps them optimize their well-being, manage their weight, and prevent or recover from lifestyle diseases. She also created the 21 Day Plant-based Health Challenge *to encourage people to go plant-based.*

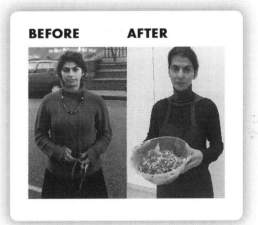

BEFORE   AFTER

Facebook: *Dr Leila D.- Plant-Powered Qi Nutrition*
Instagram: *@plantpowered_qi_nutrition or drleilad.com*

"You don't exist for half a week," had been my sister's complaint about my migraine headaches for as long as I can remember. I barely remember a time when I didn't hate the word "migraine" and its little companion, "headache."

I had my first migraine attack at the age of nine. My family was living in Iran at the time. After a few visits to doctors and undergoing necessary scans, I was diagnosed with migraine. This news didn't surprise my family. My father, two aunts and a cousin also had occasional migraines.

"She'll grow out of it," they reassured each other.

When we moved to Austria shortly after the diagnosis, my parents dragged me to more specialists, and I had more tests. Probably just the same tests as in

Iran but now under the eyes of, in my family's assumption, advanced western medicine. The tests generated the same results: all normal. The diagnosis didn't change, and the doctors couldn't offer any treatment apart from analgesic medicines to reduce the pain.

I was too young to really grasp what any of it meant. All I knew was that I'd periodically get excruciating pain on one side of my head, and I'd have to lie in a dark, quiet room until the pain subsided. I hated migraines for having taken control over my life. At school I was frequently taunted by my classmates because they'd often see me pressing my fingers into my temple and trying to shield my eyes from the light. I spent long hours lying in the school doctor's office, which meant that I was missing classes.

Looking back, I'm surprised that neither I nor my parents gave up looking for a cure. My parents took me to anybody who promised the slightest possibility of treatment. I had the weirdest treatments. One summer holiday in Iran, my uncle bought me jars of a very expensive, special kind of honey, on the advice of a holistic doctor. I was told to fast for two or three days and to drink a solution made of that honey and filtered water. I could not consume any other food or drink. It tasted awful and caused severe diarrhea. To my uncle's deep disappointment, I couldn't go through with it and quit after half a day.

My migraine attacks were debilitating. Our family doctor and my neurologist in Vienna wanted very much to help. Over the years, they prescribed any new medication that promised relief. I was never interested in learning the names of those medications, even later when I became a medical student. All I wanted was for those 'headaches' to go away. All I wanted was a normal life like the rest of the world. I had dreams and plans, so I was always on the lookout for a miracle solution.

Any book that mentioned migraine caught my attention. In one of those books, I read about a technique developed by a German doctor. I can't remember his name, but he believed that apples were the answer. I had to eat an apple every hour. Whenever in pain, the book advised the sufferers to keep eating apples until the pain subsided. My parents, probably feeling as desperate as I did, bought a big box of apples without asking any questions. For a couple of weeks, my rucksack was full of apples. Once, I even had to leave the lecture hall in a rush so that I could go and eat apples because I felt a migraine coming on. It sounds hilarious now, but it was not hilarious at the time.

Another strange treatment I tried was called "oxygen therapy." A cannula was inserted into one arm which would draw my blood and feed it into a machine. There my blood would become oxygenated and then transfused back into my body via another cannula. I had weekly "oxygen therapy" for a few months with no success. That was the most expensive and the most bizarre therapy I ever tried. When I think back to my teenage years and early university years, I'm glad there were no grave and harmful consequences from all those strange tinctures, treatments, and interventions.

Sadly, while trying to live and cope with my migraine, I developed an eating disorder. It started when I was about 13 years old. I have always had a sweet tooth and whenever I felt a headache was coming on, I ate something sweet to comfort myself. One lunchtime at school stands out in my memory. I had a headache and while waiting for the painkillers to kick in, I went to the school cafeteria and bought myself a bag of cookies. A classmate saw me wolfing down one cookie after the other and asked whether I was going to eat the whole box. I felt embarrassed and said something about the food making the pain go away.

"But you get a lot of headaches and if you continue like this, you'll put on weight," she said. Her words hurt, but not as much as the pain in my head.

Later during a visit to yet another reputable doctor I learned how not to gain weight. That doctor believed that yeast was the root of many ailments including migraines and told me to remove it from my diet. She also said that if I ever happened to eat foods containing yeast, I should just stick my finger down my throat and induce vomiting. Well-meaning advice that set me on the course of developing bulimia.

It may sound like a cliché, but the decision to become a doctor stemmed from my desire to help others, and not because I was looking for a cure for my own health issues. Studying while having to battle migraines was tough. In my first year as a medical student, I was admitted to the hospital for analgesia withdrawal and detoxification. Luckily, in Austrian medical schools attending lectures was not compulsory or I would have never been able to graduate. The regular and continuous use of analgesics and repeated vomiting led to gastritis, constipation, and other problems from overuse of headache medications. This time I didn't seek medical help. I suffered in silence. That's why I don't remember much of my fourth year of medical school. I know that I took two exams that year, but the rest is a blur to me.

Throughout the years, a few doctors had suggested that there was a psychosomatic element to my migraines, and if I were happier my migraines would vanish. It may sound peculiar, but that possibility fueled my desire to move to the United Kingdom after graduation and start afresh.

The first couple of years were great. I loved my job, especially when I started my training in pediatrics. There were even times when I was able to work despite having a migraine attack. But it wasn't long before the use of constant painkillers led to headache medication overuse.

My headaches and migraines got out of hand and took over my life. Nevertheless, I attempted to take my first medical certification exam. However, I couldn't study for it because of the frequent migraines. Finally, I decided to quit medicine. This was not an easy decision because I was giving up on my lifelong dream of being a pediatrician.

After leaving medicine, I chose a career in fitness, believing that exercise was preventive medicine. I believed that the flexibility in my new career would provide me with job satisfaction because I would have more time to focus on finding a cure for my migraines, and it would be easier to take time off whenever I had a migraine attack.

Around that time, I became vegan because of my concern for animals. I was clueless about nutrition and had no idea what I was doing. The first few months of being vegan, a junk-food vegan, I survived on peanut butter sandwiches and bland steamed vegetables. Luckily, people started asking questions about my diet. Where do I get my protein? What about soy? To answer those questions, I had to learn about nutrition.

Meanwhile, my migraines had worsened, and I now suffered from chronic headaches, which in my case meant pain 18-20 days per month, with more than 10 of them being migraine headaches. When you suffer from a chronic disease, you become tired of the constant fight and the never-ending disappointment of looking for a cure. I had reached that point. I didn't want to try new things. I was ready to give up my dreams.

Then, in 2017, my family persuaded me to try Botox injections, which were touted as the latest migraine treatment and very effective. Maybe there was still hope. I requested a referral from my family doctor. After the first round of injections at a respected migraine clinic in London, I didn't experience any change. But after the second round of injections, I noticed my condition was worse! My migraine attacks, which typically lasted two to three days at a time, now lasted five days. That was almost a whole week of my life gone! I was crushed. Not only had the Botox injections not cured my migraines, but they had increased the duration of attacks and made my life much worse.

As luck would have it, in March 2018 my sister told me about the Nutrition in Medicine Conference which was organized by the Plant-based Health Professionals UK. The talks at the one-day event blew my mind. As a doctor, I had come to believe that most cancers were a death sentence. At the conference I learned otherwise. Some people with cancers were surviving, even thriving, after converting to a whole food, plant-based diet. I wondered, if people could cure their life-threatening cancer on a whole food, plant-based diet, could such a diet address my life-long migraine attacks, as well? I left the conference with an excruciating headache, but encouraged and excited.

The idea that food could be medicine seemed too good to be true, and I was reluctant to take the plunge and change my diet. Growing up and watching my mother brew awful-smelling herbs and teas to treat colds and stomach aches, led me to believe that food had to be bad-tasting and awful-smelling to be medicinal. The thought that food could be delicious, and healing seemed absurd! But I was determined to investigate whole plant food lifestyles and started reading articles and attending webinars about them. I became inspired by the personal stories of people who overcame the greatest odds by modifying the foods they put into their bodies. I was on the edge of adopting a no-oil, whole food, plant-based diet, but couldn't quite commit.

Then, about a month after that fateful conference, I had a five-day migraine attack. Sheer desperation pushed me to change my diet overnight from a junk-food vegan diet to a no-oil, whole food, plant-based diet. The first few days were the hardest because I had a headache, but none of my comfort foods were part of the new diet. That didn't deter me though. I was determined to go through with this new diet. After the disappointing Botox injections, I knew that doctors didn't have anything more to offer.

Five days into the new diet, my ever-present headaches disappeared. I was happy, but still had misgivings because I had tried so many different treatments since age nine, that I lost track of them. Some provided relief, but only for a temporary time, never permanently. Acupuncture, for example, was the best treatment I had encountered. It gave me relief for almost a month, but then the migraines returned and no matter how many acupuncture sessions I had afterwards, the migraines did not stop. As a result, I was skeptical that anything would ever stop the migraines for good.

On the eleventh day of my new oil-free, whole food, plant-based diet, I did develop a migraine, but it was short and less intense. But no headache followed that migraine attack!

There was another appointment coming up at the migraine clinic for a third round of Botox injections. I didn't cancel it and went to share the good news with the neurologist. She asked me about my diet and said that she could never give up sugar. She then called me a "Botox success." I objected and reiterated that my migraines had gotten worse after Botox, and that it was the whole food, plant-based diet that had healed me. But she did not listen. She turned deaf to my explanation. I don't blame her. Medical schools don't teach anything about the dictum from Hippocrates: "Let food be thy medicine."

I, too, had been ignorant and oblivious to the power of food. But now that I had my life back, it was a whole new world for me, with new possibilities, new ambitions, and new dreams. I felt compelled to share the good news with people, especially fellow migraineurs. I enrolled in Dr. Colin Campbell's *Plant-based Nutrition Certificate* program at e-Cornell (part of Cornell University) to learn about plant-based diets.

The desire to help people, which had led me to choose medicine as a career, now spurred me to pursue a graduate degree in nutrition to truly understand the fundamentals of nutrition. Exactly 16 months after I adopted a no-oil, whole food plant-based diet, I was awarded a Master of Science degree with "distinction" in Clinical and Public Health Nutrition. That was a huge achievement for me. Not because I found the subject difficult or the studying to be hard, but because I never thought I'd be able to pursue and fulfil a dream. Any dream.

I have lost many years of my life and many opportunities because of my migraines. I don't like to call my migraines "a blessing in disguise," but without them I would have never learned about the power of nutrition.

Since my transition to a no-oil, whole food, plant-based lifestyle, I have averaged just two migraine days per month, down from eighteen. Occasionally, I get a five-day migraine attack, a troublesome legacy of the failed Botox injections. However, the intensity is less and I'm not bed-bound, thanks to a whole food, plant-based lifestyle.

I do still need to watch my diet. If I give in to temptation and eat vegan junk food for a couple of days in a row, I get a migraine attack. I count how many pieces of fruits and vegetables I eat. I even count the numbers of almonds, hazelnuts, or walnuts I have.

Many people call my diet extreme and time-consuming. But no food feels as good as being pain-free does. I believe that many of us have forgotten what being completely healthy feels like. We have accepted some degree of constant pains and aches as part of life and getting older. We don't realize how much time we lose every day, how much *life* we lose every day, because of being in pain and feeling fatigued.

I have been very fortunate to discover a whole food, plant-based lifestyle. It saved my life and allowed me to dream again. Now I have made it my mission to spread the message and help people suffering from chronic diseases.

To help them see the light at the end of the tunnel.

Leila Dehghan-Zaklaki, M.D.

MY REBIRTH DAY

KEN MACLEOD, PH.D.

Conditions: Cardiac arrest, heart disease, high cholesterol, high triglycerides

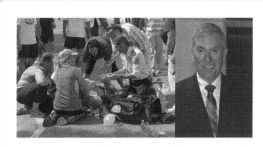

Dr. Ken MacLeod being treated during cardiac arrest/Dr. Ken MacLeod

Dr. Ken MacLeod was at the top of his career as the president of a college in Qatar. On the day set aside to celebrate National Sports Day in Qatar, with a commemorative annual 5K run, he suffered a massive cardiac arrest after finishing the race, while walking to the award presentation area. He lived to tell his story and immediately changed to a whole food, plant-based diet. Today, he is lives in Canada and is an ardent evangelist of a whole plant food lifestyle.

February 12, 2013 is the date I refer to as my *'death day'*, as opposed to my birthday. *'Rebirth day'* would be more accurate. At that time, I was President of the College of the North Atlantic-Qatar, a Canadian community college established in 2002 in the State of Qatar, a country located on the Arabian Peninsula. That rebirth day was a special day for another reason: It was National Sports Day, a national holiday in Qatar established just the year before to promote sports and healthy lifestyles in the country. In celebration of National Sports Day, the college had a full slate of sporting activities scheduled for students, faculty, and administration of the college, and for their families and public at large.

One of the activities included hosting the Terry Fox Run, an annual 5K running event that honors the courageous efforts of Canadian hero, Terry Fox, by raising funds for cancer research. Terry Fox was a remarkable Canadian athlete, humanitarian, and activist for cancer research. Despite losing a leg to cancer, Terry Fox embarked on a cross-Canada run in 1980 to raise money for cancer research. He ran 3,339 miles before succumbing to the cancer that ultimately took his life. His heroic efforts raised millions of dollars for research.

In addition to presiding over the entire day at the college, my intent was to participate in the college tennis tournament and then run in the Terry Fox Run. There were over 1,000 people on campus that day participating in various activities, many of which were family oriented, including the Terry Fox Run. I was looking forward to the run, both because it would be fun to participate in it and because at the presentations after the run, I was to introduce Judith

Fox, sister of the late Terry Fox. She had made a special trip to Qatar to attend and speak at our event.

At that time, I was 58 years old. I had always led an active lifestyle, with hockey, running, squash, and tennis being my primary sports. All my life my weight had followed a yoyo pattern; up 25 pounds or down 25 pounds usually depending on how much exercise I got. At this point, I was on the higher side of the yoyo.

It was a beautiful day in Doha, the capital of Qatar, as the days usually are. It was, however, unseasonably warm with the temperature pushing 30 degrees Celsius (86 degrees Fahrenheit).

The tennis tournament had begun the night before, and after playing in it that evening, I arrived at the campus early the next morning to continue playing doubles tennis. I expected to be finished playing tennis before the beginning of the Terry Fox Run, which began at noon. The run went without incident, and as I crossed the finish line, I caught sight of a tennis chum of mine. We walked casually along together to the presentation area.

My death day began right then.

As we walked, I had a momentary sensation that I was fainting, and everything went black. The next thing I remember is waking up in the back of an ambulance with my wife and son, a student at the College. They were sitting next to me. I was taken to the hospital, and, after several tests, I was told they were going to keep me overnight. I expressed some disappointment with that idea and said I would rather go home.

My son said, "Dad, this was pretty serious."

I replied, "People faint all the time."

He said, "Dad, you didn't faint, you had some kind of a heart attack or something else that was serious. In fact, they had to defibrillate you!."

I was shocked, literally, and figuratively!

More accurately, as I found out later at the Hamad Heart Hospital, I had had cardiac arrest, not a heart attack. Up to that point, I thought they were the same thing, but a heart attack is a circulation problem, normally caused by blockages preventing blood from flowing, and therefore preventing oxygen from getting to the heart muscles. Cardiac arrest is usually an electrical problem when the heart stops beating entirely or enters fibrillation, a superfast type of fluttering or vibration. With cardiac arrest, the threat is that the brain does not receive oxygen before brain cells begin to die. Those brain cells die very quickly, within just a few minutes without oxygen.

Coincidentally, I had attended a presentation at the college just a week before where I learned that the survival rate from an out-of-hospital cardiac arrest was about 4%. In fact, I vividly remembered the presenter putting that percentage in perspective by pointing out that in 25 cases of out-of-hospital cardiac arrests, only four people make it to the hospital, and only one walks out alive.

Little did I know less than three weeks later that one very lucky person would be me.

So, how did I survive? On that fateful day, when I had the great misfortune of having cardiac arrest, I had the tremendously good fortune to "drop dead" about 50 feet from an Emergency Medical Services team made up of five faculty members from our School of Health Sciences. There were three respiratory therapy and two paramedicine faculty members right there who had volunteered to be on duty for the Terry Fox Run.

One of them recounted later that as she rushed to give aid, she noted two things about the man lying on his back on the pavement: "It was Dr. Ken! And he was dead!"

Well, not quite. I know my faculty and how effective they are and well trained. I know that for this type of incident, I was in the best hands in Qatar. Serendipity on steroids! As I learned later, while they took turns providing CPR, a defibrillator was activated. After 'flatlining' for four minutes, the team expertly applied the paddles and gave me a shock that jolted me with a new lease on life – my heart started beating. (I was actually in cardiac fibrillation, and I have the ECG printout framed on my wall.)

In the photo of my cardiac arrest episode, I am giving a high five to the Dean of the School of Health Sciences who had joined the team. In fact, that picture was taken almost immediately after I had been defibrillated. After giving a high five, I tried to get up. The team said that my level of lucidity at that point was very odd. Since I do not remember any of it, I don't believe I was really that lucid.

While I was in the hospital, a friend gave me two books to read: *'The China Study'*, written by T. Colin Campbell, Ph.D. and Thomas M. Campbell, M.D., and *'Prevent and Reverse Heart Disease'*, by Caldwell Esselstyn, M.D. I don't know if it was my frame of mind, or the fact that these books by scientists seemed to have a credible scientific base, but I bought into both all the way.

As I was reading these two books, I had an angiogram done and discovered that I had two blockages in my coronary arteries. At this point there was quite a discussion amongst the team of cardiologists as to whether I had had cardiac arrest or a heart attack. Maybe I had a heart attack that brought on cardiac arrest, which can also happen. Regardless, the consensus was that it was indeed cardiac arrest, but the blockages now needed to be addressed. They were, with two stents. The possible recurrence of cardiac arrest was addressed with an implantable cardioverter-defibrillator or ICD, a device that is like a pacemaker with a souped-up battery to give my heart a jolt should I ever have cardiac arrest again.

I gained some level of comfort and confidence from those two procedures. But after reading those two books, I decided I had to do something more. I had to embrace veganism, fat free veganism to be exact. Or to be more precise, a whole food, plant-based (WFPB) diet. I began by searching the internet for 'fat free vegan' and clicked on the first hit on the list. I was fortunate to stumble upon Susan Voisin's excellent website, FatFreeVeganKitchen.com. I then gave my son an extensive grocery list.

Upon getting out of the hospital less than two weeks later, my life as a fat free vegan began. I have never looked back. Over seven years and counting. It helped that for the previous twenty years, I was the primary cook in the family. With a vegetarian son, I had some knowledge and expertise in cooking plant-based meals. (I liked them also, truth be told.) Now, I learned to cook fat free, whole plant food meals.

As a follow up to my incident, I had blood tests done every three months. When I entered the hospital, what I refer to as my 'overall cholesterol number' (or total cholesterol) was 7.19 or 277 (depending on which system you use), my LDL ("bad" cholesterol) was 4.06 or 157, my HDL ("good" cholesterol) was 1.20 or 46, and my triglycerides were 4.06 or 360.

On my first test, three months after my heart incident and after converting to a fat free vegan lifestyle, I had lost 35 lbs. My numbers had changed dramatically. My overall or total cholesterol was 2.79 or 108, my LDL was 1.28 or 49 (eventually it went down to 0.85 or 33), and my HDL was 1.28 or 49.

In addition to changing my diet, I was taking a prescribed statin. At this point, I asked my cardiologist to cut my medication in half. My next test, three months later, showed that my numbers had risen by a very insignificant amount. Seven years later my weight is still the same (no more yoyo, and the same weight as in high school), and my 'numbers' are still all excellent.

That said, once you have had a heart incident, monitoring, and understanding your numbers is important. Though I feel I am now in 'maintenance mode' and have truly changed my nutritional lifestyle, you can still be true to a fat-free, whole food, plant-based diet and still make mistakes. For example, early on when my numbers all plummeted, I presumed they would continue to do so and then level out. In general, they have. But on my third blood test, my triglycerides shot up to their former high!

I was flabbergasted and said to my cardiologist, "How can that happen? I religiously follow my fat-free vegan diet!" He indicated it was likely a combination of two things: portion size and eating too many starchy vegetables. I was not only not monitoring the type of vegetables I was eating, but I was eating to feel full (it is hard to drop those yoyo nutritional habits). So, I made the necessary adjustments and the impact on triglycerides was immediate. In fact, the axiom I now go by, which I had read somewhere along the way, is that it is better to live 'on the thin edge of hunger' (i.e., feeling a little hungry sometimes), than to feel stuffed.

When I tell people that I eat a vegan diet (or more accurately fat free, WFPB diet), the first thing they ask is, "Where do you get your protein?" (Many plant-based foods are high in protein, and all protein originates in plants).

They also ask, "What DO you eat?," with an implied inference that if you can't eat meat, or dairy, or foods with any degree of fat, what is there left to eat? As you may know, what we can eat with whole plant foods is a very long list, so I always answer that question by concentrating on what I can eat, rather than what I cannot eat.

In terms of cooking, I make my weekly menu management easier by having several 'go to' dishes for each mealtime: Steel cut oats with berries or CLTT (cucumber, lettuce, tomato, and tofu) sandwiches for breakfast; soups and salads for lunch; and baked tofu with veggies or kababs for dinner. I also prepare dishes that I can freeze and thaw to eat at any time. Veggie chili is a good example of the latter. Then, I add to that list from the plethora of plant-based websites available on the internet. I figure out how to make dishes that normally contain meat, dairy, or animal fat, without those ingredients and still taste delicious. Dinner guests are amazed how good my chana masala and tofu 'butter' curry taste (without a cup of butter ghee in each), and my tofu kebabs with various fat free bastings. My black bean burgers (thanks to Susan Voisin) are always a hit at a BBQ.

With the type of heart incident I had, and the cardio stats before and after the incident (and my conversion to a whole plant food diet), I am not only fortunate to have survived and recovered, but I truly believe I am healthier now than I was before. In fact, I have never had a symptom of a heart problem, neither before nor after my incident. Given that, my doctors advised me, once I was fully recovered, to go back and do whatever physical activities I was doing before my incident. So, the following year, on National Sports Day, I played again in the college tennis tournament, and again ran the Terry Fox Run. Talk about tempting fate! I finally got to introduce Judith Fox. In doing so, I exclaimed, "I have been dying to introduce Judith!."

Now I am retired and back in Canada. I have become a fat free, plant-based, whole food evangelist to anyone who will listen. That is why I wrote my story for *Forks Over Knives*. This is why I wrote my story for this book.

I believe it is the right thing to do for my body, for people, for animals, and for the planet. I am the living proof that it works – emphasis on the word, *living*.

Ken MacLeod, Ph.D.

OTHER STORIES OF DISEASE REVERSAL
BY DAN PURJES

Many people whom we, the authors, know, with many different chronic diseases reversed their disease by converting to a whole plant food lifestyle. For one reason or another, some of these people did not write their story for this book. Since their chronic ailments are known to cause suffering to millions of people, we thought it worth describing what happened after they converted to a whole plant food diet.

Since they did not write a story for our book in their own first person voice, I provide a synopsis of their story written by me in the third person in this section. To maintain confidentiality only a first name has been provided and that, too, has been changed. Most personal details have not been disclosed to increase confidentiality. Each of the people in this section are personally known to us or to the physician (or other person) who told us about them. Each of these people may have suffered from multiple chronic diseases. I highlighted the one or two that I think have the greatest impact, either because they apply to a great many people or because they are somewhat unique.

The takeaway here, as with all the stories in this book, is that the underlying cause of almost all chronic diseases are the toxic foods we consume multiple times every day. When these unhealthy foods are eliminated from the daily diet, the body immediately begins to heal itself.

Sometimes that healing process can completely reverse a chronic disease. Not only does the person feel healthy with no symptoms, and ceases to take any medications, but there are no markers in the body indicating the presence of disease. Other times, the disease has already caused such significant damage to the body over a long period that it is not possible to completely reverse the disease. But in all cases, healing begins almost immediately upon conversion to a whole food, plant-based lifestyle, and the person will find themselves feeling much better within days or weeks.

It's that fast.

If you don't believe it, try it for just 30 days. See how much better you feel right away!

Dan Purjes

DIVERTICULITIS

James was a lively, engaging real estate broker in his mid-forties who had diverticulitis when we met. My wife and I had asked him to show us a number of real estate properties in a new community to which we were considering moving. As we drove off from his office to view some homes, I asked James questions about the community and what drew him to relocate. Naturally, that involved him telling us about his life – a topic most people like to speak about. In the midst of this, I asked James about his health. That is something I do with most people I meet because I always want to deliver the message of whole plant food living and how it dramatically improves life.

James certainly appeared outwardly healthy. He was trim and fit, with a bounce to his step and a sparkle in his eyes. But he had diverticulitis – inflammation of the intestine. From time to time he experienced flare-ups that caused severe pain or discomfort, preventing him from eating nuts, seeds and certain fruits such as berries that contain seeds. Most people who suffer from diverticulitis are advised by their physicians to avoid nuts, seeds, berries and certain other foods, in the mistaken belief that they can get trapped in pockets of the intestines, thereby causing inflammation and infection. This theory has recently been disproven. In certain cases, the disease can cause significant inflammation and damage to the body and can even be fatal.

As with many chronic diseases today, physicians don't understand what causes diverticulitis. There are suggestions that genes play a role, or not enough fiber in the diet, or too much animal-based foods, or very dense food such as nuts and seeds that get trapped in the intestines, along with other theories. But nothing has been proven conclusively in scientific studies.

However, I have known several people to reverse their diverticulitis by converting to a whole food, plant-based diet. James was one of them.

I often share with the people suffering from diverticulitis how the diet they've been eating for years has wreaked havoc on their body. All animal foods and refined foods increase chronic inflammation, which has devastating consequences on the body. (In addition, there are other lifestyle insults such as stress, pollution, drugs, alcohol, smoking, etc.). I tell them that chronic inflammation manifests in damage to one or more organs. In James' case, the organ that was injured was his intestines.

The primary problem is not the nuts, seeds or berries that he eats. The problem is the diet of meat, dairy, and processed foods that caused the initial injury and secondary inflammation. Nuts and seeds then get lodged in intestines that are already inflamed.

I explain that the body has an enormous ability to heal as soon as these insults are eliminated, especially those related to diet. Almost all of these people say they never knew that their diet could be so harmful. Some of these people are physicians, who are not taught about nutrition in medical school nor in post-graduate training. They did not know Hippocrates' dictum, "Let food be thy medicine." In fact, one of these physicians told me, "You know more about nutrition, Dan, than most physicians!"

These people were not aware of the harmful consequences of a diet composed of animal-based food products, packaged foods, and of large amounts of oil and fats. When they express skepticism that changing their diet can heal their disease, I suggest they try it for 30 days and see what happens.

"What have you got to lose?" I ask, "except your diverticulitis?"

That often hooks them.

James decided right then and there, on our way to the next home showing, to immediately convert to a whole plant food diet.

"If I can eat the foods I love and miss so much, like berries, nuts and seeds," he said, "it will be worth it! If I can avoid having the pain and discomfort in my gut, and not having to run to the bathroom or take pills, it's worth it."

Three weeks later, James called me. He was very excited. It was only three weeks, not even a month, yet he was already eating nuts, seeds and berries without a problem. He couldn't believe it!

He also told me he had not felt this good and healthy since his teenage years. He had more energy than ever, fewer aches and pains, and no bowel irregularity. He had convinced his wife to join him, and now even his kids were interested.

My wife and I ended up buying a new home through James, and we love it and our new community. I asked James to write his story for this book. He said he would, but after waiting over two years for it, I decided to write it for him and include it in this section. I believe it is important for others who endure this painful disease to read his story.

THE PROJECTIONIST

A projectionist in one of the movie theaters where Eating You Alive, the film of which I was the Executive Producer, was screened wrote an amazing letter to the filmmakers. She wrote she had been so moved by the film she was projecting, that she decided to immediately convert to the whole plant food diet described in the film. She lost 100 pounds in 8 months and has a new life of health.

We never met this projectionist. She was in the projection booth of the theater the whole time. She wrote to us out of the blue.

OBESITY NIGHTMARE

There are many stories in this book about obesity because so many people struggle with weight. In fact, about 75% or more of the stories involve someone who is overweight. In the USA, about three out of four people are overweight, and many are severely overweight. Clinically and morbidly overweight.

The obesity epidemic has prompted the authors of this book to follow it up with a new book currently in the works called, OBESITY REVERSAL HOPE! Real Stories by Real People. This book will be published in the first half of 2022.

Much of the time, when someone converts to a whole food, plant based diet, they lose weight rapidly. Time and again, the authors of this book have heard people say that the weight melted off them, no matter how much they ate, as long as it was the right foods.

However, there are people for whom weight loss is especially difficult. There are several possible reasons for this, but the fact is that if a person fastidiously follows a whole plant food diet, with no oils, processed foods, or excess plant based fats, they will definitely lose weight, and lots of it. When people fail to lose weight on a whole foods, plant-based diet with no oils and minimal fats it is usually because they are eating junk vegan food, or highly processed vegan food with lots of vegetable oil. Veggie burgers, French fries, and salads with lots of dressing are all plant-based, but they are loaded with oils that will add to weight. The story below is not about one particular person. Instead it is a compendium of several stories of different people who struggled long and hard with excess weight until they found their way to such a diet. None of these people would write their story for this book for one reason or another, so I combined them into one story since they were so similar.

Angelina (not a real person, but a made-up name for this amalgamation of several women) had ballooned up to 290 pounds after the birth of her children. She liked to believe that it was pregnancy weight gain, but deep down she knew the truth was that she had struggled with weight as far back as she could remember, all the way back to grammar school.

Angelina grew up on a dairy farm. There was always lots of milk, cheese and butter on the table. Plenty of eggs for breakfast, and chicken or beef the rest of the day. Like many American families, her parents knew nothing about healthy nutrition. At home and in school, she ate unhealthy meals loaded with fat, sugar and salt. As a young child, Angelina started gaining weight, and this continued throughout her adolescent and teenage years. When she graduated high school, she was obese and miserable.

She tried every diet out there, but the results were always the same. While she was on a diet, she would lose some weight, yet never enough and never for long. When she could no longer continue on the diet she, the weight came roaring back, sometimes more than before. She tried unusual ways to lose weight like restricting her diet to just one type of food such as potatoes or grapefruit. She tried a vegetarian diet, juice diets, intermittent fasting, diet pills, acupuncture and hypnosis. Doctors prescribed various drugs and strange remedies. But her weight just kept going up. She did not want to have bariatric surgery because she heard that 25% of them failed, and even the ones that were successful often required a re-do after a few years.

Not only did Angelina's weight continue to increase, but she began suffering the consequences of carrying lots of excess weight , including pain in her joints, chronic fatigue, and brain fog. Additionally, she developed Type 2 diabetes along with a leaky gut and fatty liver disease. Angelina became more and more depressed as her weight grew to almost 300 pounds and her future seemed hopeless.

Then she discovered the whole plant food lifestyle through a friend who recommended she read several books about plant-based nutrition. She was not sure this would be the answer, and she found the thought of giving up her beloved dairy and cheese almost impossible to imagine. But she was so desperate she was ready to try anything.

To her surprise, she found plant-based meals to be colorful and delicious. She had worried about getting enough protein, but that did not seem to be a problem once she learned how much protein is available in a plant-based diet. Even giving up dairy was not as traumatic as she had feared. After a few weeks, she found she did not miss dairy. After a few months on a whole foods, plant-based diet, she was amazed to find that dairy, especially melted cheese, actually nauseated her. The brain fog began to lift and her A1c level (a blood marker for diabetes) began to come down. But even though she lost weight it was not that much.

As Angelina read more books about plant-based lifestyles, and as she watched plant-based documentaries, it dawned on her that she was still consuming too many processed foods, and too much fat and oil. Even though these were plant-based, they were not that nutritious and they were keeping her from losing weight. When she finally cut them out of her diet, she lost weight. And lots of it.

Combining her new plant-based diet with vigorous exercise brought about the weight loss she had always wanted. Over a two-year period, Angelina lost 150 pounds — over half her body weight! She also lost her diabetes and other ailments. And she was no longer depressed, because she now had a whole new life.

RHEUMATOID ARTHRITIS (RA)
RA STORY #1: A PHYSICIAN WITH RHEUMATOID ARTHRITIS

Dr. Joshua, "Doc Josh" as he was called, was a celebrity doctor. He had graduated from one of the finest medical schools in the USA and had gone on to do his residency at a major university hospital. His father was a renowned physician, and Doc Josh was following in his footsteps.

But after 10 years of practice at the hospital, Doc Josh wanted more. He had been the "house doctor" for a popular TV program, where he answered medical questions that came up during the show. He was handsome and smart, and he liked the attention he was getting from the TV show. An opportunity came his way to host another TV program, and he jumped on it. He was also getting lots of speaking engagements from his increasing popularity, and he began writing books that were well received.

As time went on, his days were so hectic he could barely find time to eat. Like many busy people, Doc Josh resorted to pizza and soda for lunch, fast food burgers, French fries, or other take-out and fast food for his regular meals. Though he had been vain about his once muscular body, he was putting on pounds rapidly. He was at least 30 pounds too heavy.

Then the pain came. Aching joints, fatigue, stiffness, inflammation, and other symptoms. Doc Josh was diagnosed with rheumatoid arthritis. He was prescribed the usual medications for autoimmune diseases. A chemotherapy drug to suppress his immune system and steroids for the inflammation. The side effects were terrible. He even had surgery to alleviate the havoc the disease was causing on certain joints.

When I met him, I told Doc Josh there was a better way. A way without drugs and without side effects. He was amazed to hear that a whole food, plant based diet could reverse his disease. He had never learned about nutrition in medical school or heard of it during medical residency. He could not believe that nutrition was all that was needed to reverse chronic disease. He had always held the belief that chronic disease could never be reversed.

I introduced him to a plant-based physician I knew who put him on a 6-week program of raw, whole plant foods. In less than a month his symptoms cleared up. He was so amazed by this that he spoke of it on TV shows he was on. In fact, he introduced this plant-based physician to a national TV audience as his savior.

In addition to losing his rheumatoid arthritis, Doc Josh was thrilled to lose his excess weight. In just a few weeks, he was back to a trim weight.

I asked Doc Josh to write a story for this book, but I could never get him to do that. For one thing, he was way too busy. Another reason was that he eventually went back to his prior eating habits . This was because his days were so hectic, he said, with more engagements that he could not find the time to prepare whole plant food meals. So, he started eating pizza and fast foods again.

Of course, his rheumatoid arthritis came roaring back.

I plan to send him a copy of this book so he can reclaim his health once again, perhaps sharing his own version of his story in a future book

RA STORY #2: A BANK PRESIDENT WITH RHEUMATOID ARTHRITIS

Bob was the retired president of a bank. I had gotten to know him well years earlier, but had not seen him for a while when we got together in a café. I said as we sat down, "You don't look so good, Bob."

"I don't feel so good, Dan," he replied.

I asked him to tell me why. As he described his symptoms, I interrupted and said, "It sounds like you have rheumatoid arthritis."

Bob said that's exactly what he had. He was quite depressed about it. Not only did he have aches and pains in many joints, but he was always fatigued. He didn't even have enough energy to complete 18 rounds of golf. That's terrible for a banker.

I told Bob he could reverse his rheumatoid arthritis in a short time by converting to a whole foods, plant based diet. I knew of that happening with many people. He found that hard to believe but he was willing to try anything to get healthy. I introduced him to a plant-based physician I knew very well who then put Bob on a nutrient-rich, plant-based diet.

Three weeks later, Bob called me with unmistakable delight in his voice. Not only were his aches and pains gone, not only had the fatigue disappeared, not only was he off all medications, but he was playing 18 holes of golf again with lots of energy and enthusiasm. He couldn't believe that it was due to being on a whole plant food diet for just three weeks. After many miserable years of suffering, it seemed miraculous to be cured in only 3 weeks!

ROCKS IN HER EYES

Anne is a dear friend of my wife's. She visits us once or twice a year even though she lives hundreds of miles away. During one visit, she complained about several ailments including being overweight and having no energy. Other problems included constipation, high blood pressure, insomnia, and more. I encouraged her to try a whole plant food diet for just a few weeks and see what it would do for her.

Six week later, Anne emailed me that the plant-based diet had done wonders for her. In addition to losing weight and having way more energy, she said the "rocks in her eyes" were shrinking, something she never thought would happen.

Rocks in the eyes? I had never heard of it before. My ophthalmologist explained this was the colloquial term for a condition where certain minerals coagulate in the eyeball and form dense granules that obstruct vision. There is no cure or effective treatment for this condition, and the ophthalmologist had never heard of it reversing, but that was what was happening to Anne. She was amazed and so was I. So was the ophthalmologist.

I asked Anne to write her story for this book, but she never got around to it.

VERTIGO

Linda was with me when she had a severe vertigo attack. Linda was in her 60s and retired. She was also a close friend of my wife's. We were in my telescope observatory – a silo-like structure with a rotating dome on top. Perhaps it was the confines of an unusual round room that triggered the attack. Perhaps it was something else. In any case, I had to call other people for help get Linda to bed. Even in bed, she complained the room was still spinning, and she felt very nauseous.

This was not Linda's first vertigo attack. She had them often, and they were getting more frequent and more intense. Linda was also quite overweight with other health issues. However, the vertigo was the worst issue. It prevented her from having any semblance of a normal life. She couldn't drive or engage in any activities that might prove dangerous to herself or others because she could never tell when a vertigo attack might come on. She sought help from numerous physicians, clinics and hospitals, but there was no relief. There were many treatments, including pharmaceuticals and being swung upside down for long periods of time in a specially designed frame, but these methodologies did not work.

I had tried to persuade Linda to try a whole plant food diet. There was no assurance that would help her vertigo, but it wouldn't hurt to try, and there could be improvement in her other ailments. But Linda resisted because she did not want to give up her animal-based foods.

Linda was a close friend of Anne's (see the above story, "Rocks in Her Eyes"). When Anne sent me the email marveling at how the "rocks in her eyes" were shrinking, I asked her if I could forward the email to Linda, in an effort to encourage Linda to try a whole plant food diet. Anne said, "Sure. Go right ahead."

Anne's email did the trick. Linda went on a plant-based diet. But I did not know about it until much later. Several months went by before Linda sent me an email saying that converting to a plant-based diet had greatly improved her vertigo condition. In fact, she had not had an episode in months. She was incredulous that a change in diet could accomplish what none of the hospitals, clinics and medical practices, drugs and upside down contraptions, could accomplish.

I asked Linda to write her story for this book. She attempted to, but it was not written very well. She eventually went back to animal-based foods because she found them so comforting. In no time, her vertigo came back. She asked us not to publish her story. We didn't.

However, vertigo affects millions of people, especially as they age, and there is often no effective, long-lasting treatment. We felt it important to tell Linda's story to show how a whole plant food diet could help vertigo.

Here is a paraphrased and heavily edited excerpt from Linda's own story: "I have not had a vertigo attack in the six months since converting to a plant-based diet. I also experienced other important benefits. My heartburn is gone and my cholesterol dropped a whopping 100 points! I am now living a somewhat normal life in that I am driving and socializing."

There are a number of possible causes of vertigo, several of which are surely connected to diet. Vertigo is known to involve inflammation of certain structures in the inner ear and eustachian tubes. A whole foods plant based diet is known to reduce inflammation, whereas refined, processed and animal based foods are known to increase inflammation.

PARKINSON'S DISEASE

My friend, Marcus, came down with Parkinson's disease several years ago. It has been terrible to witness his physical and mental deterioration over time. It keeps getting worse and worse. Although he takes medications to reduce the tremors in his hands and legs, they are still quite noticeable. His cognitive abilities and memory continue to decline.. He moves slowly and stiffly, and is quite lethargic. He nods off often at a meal or sitting in his living room when we listen to music together or just talk.

One of our favorite activities was to listen to all kinds of music on his high-end audio system. We still do that but not as much anymore. Everything gets more and more difficult with this disease. He has to keep increasing the medications to control the tremors and other symptoms. The more medications he takes, the more he zones out.

Marcus was one of those guys who was always in the gym, working out for two or more hours every day. His body resembled that of a Greek statue and he was an excellent athlete. He was very proud of his chiseled body. He was not bulky, just very well defined. He did a lot of aerobic exercises including running and playing tennis.

Marcus thought of himself as being very healthy. But his diet was the typical macho Western diet favored by most bodybuilders – lots of animal-based foods high in protein and very little in the way of whole plant foods and whole grains. He leaned towards the type of diet sometimes known as the "caveman" or keto diet.

Marcus knew that I was on a whole plant food diet, and to be frank, he thought that was ridiculous. Surely, I was not getting enough protein, in his view. I did not have the muscles or body build that he had, but he could see I was healthy. As his Parkinson's disease continued to worsen, he asked if I thought a whole plant food diet could help.

I told him it might be because Parkinson's disease has a strong inflammatory component, and lots of scientific research has demonstrated that animal-based foods and processed foods are highly inflammatory, whereas whole plant foods are anti-inflammatory and actually help lower chronic inflammation.

"Why don't you try it for a few weeks and see how you feel?" I asked him. "What have you got to lose, except maybe some of your symptoms?"

I could find no research on how a whole foods, plant-based diet impacts Parkinson's disease, but it certainly couldn't hurt and would likely improve his overall health, at the very least.

I told this to Marcus over lunch at a diner, while he had his usual cheeseburger and fries. I had a salad. He pushed his cheeseburger aside and decided right then and there to try a whole plant food diet.

Later, I explained to Marcus and his wife the basics of a whole plant food lifestyle. I emphasized that his best chance of success depended on his wife also adopting a whole plant food diet to support her husband. Unfortunately, she did not do that.

Three weeks later, I got a phone call from a friend we had in common, also a music and audio enthusiast named Donald, who was aware that Marcus had switched to a whole plant food diet to improve his Parkinson's disease. Donald said he couldn't believe how much "smoother" Marcus looked. I was confused and asked him what he meant by "smoother"?

Donald said, "His tremors are much less. His hands and legs don't shake as much. He seems much more alert and present. He's not falling asleep when we listen to music."

A few days later, Marcus' wife came to our home, brimming with joy that her husband seemed to be so much better. In fact, she told me and my wife that he had reduced his medication in half, with the approval of his physician, yet his condition continued to improve. This was encouraging news after only a few weeks on the plant-based diet.

I became excited at the possibility that there might be a new and productive way to deal with Parkinson's disease. The best of the current treatment regimens for Parkinson's disease only slow down the progression of the disease, but do not stop the progression or reverse it.

Regrettably, Marcus abandoned the whole plant food diet a few days later, and his condition rapidly deteriorated back to what it had been. He craved animal-based foods too much, he said, and he could not give them up. Donald then told me that Marcus had lost his "smoothness" and the tremors were noticeably worse. He was no longer as alert. Marcus' wife said the same. It was all so sad.

Just recently, though, Marcus announced he would try the whole plant food diet again. I do hope he sticks with it. He could be a beacon of hope for others suffering from Parkinson's disease.

BONES AND JOINT REPLACEMENT

Liam is an orthopedic surgeon who is plant-based. He had reached out to me to ask for help in forming a new, plant-based, non-profit organization dedicated to teaching the benefits of whole plant food diets to people in our community. At our plant-based, dinner, I asked him how he came to be plant-based.

"That's easy," said Liam. "The orthopedic surgeons in our large clinic, including myself, perform hundreds of surgeries a year, repairing bone fractures and replacing joints. We observed that patients on a whole food, plant-based diet heal much faster and stronger than those on an animal-based diet and processed foods."

Liam continued, "That's what got me and some of my physician partners to investigate this further. We were amazed by what we found. Countries that consume lots of dairy per person, such as the US and the UK, have the highest rates of bone fractures and joint replacements, whereas countries that consume the least amount of dairy per person, such as Japan and Korea, have the lowest rates of fractures and joint replacements. This is the complete opposite of what you'd expect to find according to the dairy industry. It's the complete opposite of their marketing campaign, 'Milk builds strong bones', isn't it?"

Liam then hit me with a stunning statement. "In fact, we came to realize that in the thousands of joint replacements we had done, we never did one in a plant-based person unless it was due to trauma. Their bones and joints don't degenerate the way they do in animal-based people. We find that bones in people on animal-based diets are much worse."

Liam explained further, "Most of the joint replacements we did in animal food-based patients was due to deterioration of their joints from wear and tear. You can actually see and feel how bones and cartilage in animal-based people turn mushy or brittle with age, and they easily break. That doesn't seem to happen to plant-based people."

He concluded by saying, "That's what convinced me to switch to a whole plant food lifestyle, myself. I've never been happier, and I want to spread the message beyond my patients to the rest of the people in our community."

CARDIOLOGIST WITH A HEART

One day, while hiking up a hill with one of my friends who is also my cardiologist, I noticed he was huffing and puffing. We are both about the same age. I pointed out to him that I was the patient who had a heart attack and he was the doctor who had put a stent into me, yet he was short of breath and I was not. Could it be that my becoming plant-based had improved my health to a greater extent than his?

When my cardiologist saw the dramatic improvement in my laboratory and clinical data after switching to a whole plant-food lifestyle – improvements in cholesterol, triglycerides, blood pressure, chronic inflammation and other markers – he decided to convert as well. He did not convert 100%, but even the 80% conversion he claimed resulted in great benefits. He lost 20 pounds, and his cholesterol fell markedly, while other biomarkers improved significantly. Every time I went to his office he would take out a small piece of paper and proudly show me his latest, improving biomarkers.

And the next time we hiked up the hill, he was not short of breath.

The following story "bites"
were forwarded to us by
Joel Fuhrman, M.D., the internationally
renowned physician and author of many books
including the bestselling, Eat To Live.

SUCCESS STORIES FOR DAN PURJES AND DR. SCOTT STOLL

BY JOEL FUHRMAN, M.D.

NAME: Cassie and Dave

HEALTH PROBLEMS: Food addiction, overweight, migraines, brain fog, lack of energy, constant sinus infections and more.

Weight:
Cassie Before: 162 pounds
Cassie After: 111 pounds

Dave Before: 250 pounds
Dave After: 145 pounds

Although they were only in their late 40s, Cassie and Dave felt old, unhealthy and tired. This married couple shared indigestion, back pain, and eczema. They would both develop frequent and even chronic sinus infections. They knew they were food addicts and were troubled by it. Their toxic lifestyle was taking a terrible toll.

Upon discovering Dr. Fuhrman's diet recommendations, centered on nutrient-dense, whole plant foods, the science resonated with them. Cassie and Dave were driven by a deep passion to get healthy and change their lives for the better. The understanding and control Dr. Fuhrman's program gave them over their cravings and addictions even empowered Dave to stop smoking.

Cassie and Dave have undergone what they call "an amazing" physical and mental transformation. Neither one has suffered from a sinus infection since starting the program, and both report that their headaches are gone. They both run and hike at least 20 miles a week. Their children have also made healthier changes to their own diets and now feel better, too.

NAME: Kate

HEALTH PROBLEMS: Pernicious anemia, overweight, high cholesterol, lack of energy.

Weight:
Before: 170 pounds
After: 106 pounds

Kate couldn't work, had zero energy, and was diagnosed with pernicious anemia, as well as a non-specific autoimmune disease with heightened markers of inflammation. She took the prescribed vitamin B12, but it did not help her fatigue and she had to quit her job. Then she found Dr. Fuhrman's nutrient-dense, whole plant-food eating approach, and she realized that her diet was the cause of her ailments.

Both Kate and her husband committed 100% to Dr. Fuhrman's diet. Now Kate has boundless energy and has no markers of autoimmune disease. Her cholesterol went from 239 to 129. She feels "back in the land of the living" and feels lucky to have found the answer through Dr. Fuhrman to excellent health.

NAME: Debra

HEALTH PROBLEM: Lupus

Debra suffered from Lupus for 20 years. She took many drugs, including Plaquenil, Methotrexate and Prednisone in increasing dosages, and she lived isolated and in pain for decades.

While searching for help, she tried acupuncture, chiropractic, herbs, supplements, antibiotics and other treatments without success.

After discovering Dr. Fuhrman's nutrient-dense, whole plant-food program, she made a complete recovery from Lupus, and now lives a normal life, a life full of energy and without medications or joint pain.

A HEART ATTACK WAS THE BEST THING THAT HAPPENED TO ME

BY DAN PURJES

Conditions: Heart disease, overweight, trigger finger, gingivitis, periodontal disease

Dan Purjes is one of the authors of this book. He became vegetarian at age 18 due to concerns about health and animals. But he did not discover a whole foods, plant-based (WFPB) lifestyle until after he had a heart attack at age 61. It changed his life.

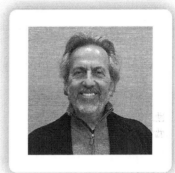

As Dan continued down the WFPB road, he met and spoke with many plant-based physicians and their patients, and read research articles and books on plant-based nutrition. As his health continued to flourish from a plant-based diet, Dan decided to commit himself to promoting the ability of such a lifestyle to reverse and prevent the myriad diseases that afflict humanity today. That led to the idea of compiling a book of stories told by people who had reversed chronic diseases through conversion to a WFPB lifestyle. Although such stories can be found in many places on the Internet and in print, there was no one book that provided a group of stories about different diseases. Dan took the idea to his friend, Dr. Scott Stoll, who promptly agreed to co-author the book. Dan and his wife, Edna ("Ed"), have funded plant-based scientific studies at major university hospitals. Dan joined the boards of several non-profit organizations promoting the benefits of plant-based health. He funded and was the Executive Producer for two films focused on plant-based health: Eating You Alive, *and* DISEASE REVERSAL HOPE: The Film. *Dan also co-founded and helped fund the launch of the International Journal of Disease Reversal & Prevention, the world's first peer-reviewed medical journal dedicated to disease reversal, and also the Disease Reversal & Prevention Digest.*

Dan's work has been going on for several years. But it is just the beginning.

In December 2011, I had a heart attack.

It was one of the best things that ever happened to me.

I had gone skiing that day at Alta Ski Area in Utah. It was at an elevation of almost 11,000 feet. The higher the elevation, the thinner the atmosphere and oxygen, and the greater the stress on the heart.

I did not feel anything adverse during that day of skiing, but around 2 AM I woke up with a sharp pain in the middle of my chest. Heart disease was rampant on both sides of my family and I knew I was at risk for the disease, so naturally I wondered if this could be a heart attack. But there were no other indications of a heart attack – no palpitations, no pain elsewhere, no sweats, nothing – and the pain went away after about 20 minutes, so I put it down to indigestion. I went skiing again the next day.

The pain came back again in the middle of the following night, like before. Again, I had no other symptoms of heart distress so I thought perhaps it was another bout of indigestion. I almost never take drugs, but this night I took a Prilosec to see if it would help. The pain went away again. I figured it was indigestion that Prilosec subdued.

The third day, I went snowshoeing uphill for 3 miles. I can be stubbornly stupid in my denials. This time, the pain came on quickly and I knew it had to be cardiac related. I immediately went to the hospital ER. They confirmed a heart attack and admitted me to the hospital. The following day I was taken to the catheterization lab for angioplasty.

While recuperating in the Intensive Care Unit following the angioplasty and a stent insertion, I saw an interview of Bill Clinton on CNN that changed my life. President Clinton had lost 30 pounds in 90 days. He explained that this was because he had been suffering from angina chest pain, even though he had undergone quadruple bypass surgery a few years earlier, after leaving the White House. His cardiologist said there was nothing that could be done for him, and his options were limited. Clinton refused to accept this and searched for other options. He came across the landmark book, *Prevent and Reverse Heart Disease,* by Caldwell Esselstyn, Jr., M.D.

Dr. Esselstyn demonstrated vividly in his book through many cardiac images how cardiovascular disease can be dramatically reversed through a whole foods, plant-based (WFPB) diet. President Clinton went on the diet, lost 30 pounds, and said the he hadn't felt so good since being a teenager. And I'm watching this on the TV in the ICU.

I had been a vegetarian almost my entire life. I mistakenly believed that being vegetarian was all the protection I needed against heart disease. But I was not WFPB. I ate lots of dairy, eggs, and processed packaged foods. That's what did me in.

The hospital I was in had no vegetarian items on the menu. My wife had left the hospital to buy vegetarian food for me. While she was out, I saw the interview of Bill Clinton on CNN. I called my wife and said, "Forget the food. Get the book!" She returned to the hospital with Dr. Esselstyn's book and we read it together that night. By morning we had both converted to a WFPB lifestyle.

Within six weeks, I lost over 20 pounds. My cholesterol dropped from 215 (red zone) to 147 ("heart attack proof" zone), my LDL ('bad") cholesterol fell from 140 to 94, my C-Reactive Protein (CRP), a key marker of inflammation, fell from 3.4 (high risk for cardiovascular event) to 0.6 (low risk for cardiovascular event), and my blood pressure fell by 20 points. I went off all medications, and I felt terrific.

The transformation in my health is amazing. I ski expert runs at 11,000 foot elevations for hours with no issues. When I return to the locker room at the end of a powder ski day, I hear lots of moaning from my fellow locker room denizens about sore muscles and joints. Skiers who are much younger than me are popping ibuprofen like it's candy, or taking multiple shots of alcohol to ease their pain. I don't need or want them.

I hike and bike, kayak for miles, and work out in the gym an hour or more with no problems. I don't mean to suggest that my heart is in great shape. It's not. My heart attack destroyed important heart muscle and it will never regenerate. My ejection fraction (a measure of heart pumping efficiency) is below normal and will never recover to normal levels. When I ski or bike, I have to stop more often and rest. But it's not a big deal. I'm living a full, active and joyful life.

I find I have lots of energy, and almost never get headaches, stomach aches, or aches of any kind. I rarely get sick. I did have COVID-19 at the end of 2020, before vaccinations were generally available. I was sick with fever, body aches and fatigue, but no other symptoms. It was quite mild and lasted only two days. Six months later, research was published in the British Medical Journal that doctors on a plant-based diet, who were front-line Covid workers, were 73% less likely to get moderate to severe Covid. I believe it! I believe it through my own actual experience.

I have found other interesting health improvements. Sometimes, these health improvements ease into my body almost without notice. For example, I used to suffer from a condition called stenosing tenosynovitis, commonly known as "trigger finger". This causes fingers to lock in a bent position, which is quite painful. I had to straighten my finger with my other hand, snapping it straight quite painfully. This occurs when inflammation narrows the space within the sheath that surrounds the tendon of the affected finger. It often happens when lifting heavy items by a handle, like a suitcase.

The most common treatments for trigger finger are anti-inflammatory drugs, including steroids, or surgery. Recently, it dawned on me that I had not had a trigger finger episode in years, not since converting to a WFPB lifestyle. That would make sense because such a lifestyle is known to reduce inflammation throughout the body. I didn't take note of it before because the trigger finger in my case was an occasional occurrence, not continuous. How wonderful not to suffer from it anymore!

Another improvement relates to pollen. I would get hay fever or allergic reactions to pollen every spring and fall. Now, no more. Also, no periodontal disease. I no longer suffer from it, (See my 2nd story, immediately following this one.)

Life is good! So very good.

It can be like that for everyone. All that's needed is to be open to fully adopting a WFPB lifestyle. Try it for 90 days and you'll never go back – back to animal-based foods, back to processed junk foods, back to the days of misery.

Dan Purjes

REVERSING PERIODONTAL DISEASE

BY DAN PURJES

Conditions: Periodontal disease, gingivitis

All the stories in this book tell the tales of people who have reversed one or more chronic diseases by converting to a whole plant food diet. But there are other natural ways of reversing and preventing chronic diseases. I'd like to describe how I reversed periodontal disease – gingivitis and periodontitis – naturally. This did not happen due to conversion to a whole plant food diet, though when I did convert years later my gums and teeth stayed healthy. It happened due to a natural hygienic process.

I grew up in a family that never placed much emphasis on oral hygiene. Consequently, I did not floss or brush my teeth regularly, I did not go for dental cleanings, and I did not take care of my mouth. Going to the dentist was something I always avoided. What kid wants to brush their teeth or go to the dentist if they don't have to? Not me.

By the time I was 30, I had serious dental problems. I lost a tooth, an important molar, to decay and gum disease. When I went to the dentist because I could no longer ignore the pain in my mouth, he told me I had an abscess and a deep pocket. The molar could not be saved and had to be extracted. A bridge and fake tooth was installed.

Then he shocked me further by telling me that at the rate I was going, I would lose most of my teeth by the time I was in my 60s. He told me I had severe periodontitis. My gums were inflamed, they bled frequently and easily, and the pockets around my teeth were unnaturally deep. He told me I had the mouth of someone twice my age. If I didn't start taking care of my teeth and gums right away, I would surely lose my teeth.

Periodontal disease, or periodontitis, is inflammation of the gums. It leads to destruction of tissue both on the outside and inside of the gums. (Gingivitis is an early and milder form of periodontal disease and can often be reversed through proper dental hygiene without the need for gum surgery.) As periodontitis advances, and bacteria destroy the gum tissue, they also attack the teeth themselves. Pockets form inside the gums and the teeth begin to loosen as there is less tissue surrounding and supporting the teeth. Painful abscesses can develop that further weaken the dental structure. Eventually, the teeth fall out. Periodontal disease can also lead to erosion and destruction of the jawbone. Then, even implants can be difficult. The further periodontal disease advances, the more pain, suffering and cost is involved in trying to remedy it.

I decided I had to do something about my periodontal disease. Someone told me about a new approach to periodontitis developed by a dentist named Dr. Paul Keyes who was a dental researcher at the National Institutes of Health.

I went to the local library and asked to see whatever dental and periodontal journals they had. (This was in the early 1980s, in the days before the Internet.) I sat in the library for hours on end reading these journals.

Dr. Keyes had published peer-reviewed articles on his research, which delved into the cause of periodontal disease. He focused on the anaerobic bacteria found under the gums and on the gum line. He demonstrated that these were the culprits behind periodontal disease. Dr. Keyes devised a treatment methodology centered on using hydrogen peroxide and baking soda that were inimical to these bacteria, as well as bactericides that attacked them.

This made a lot of sense to me. His research and treatment methods caused a great deal of angst in the periodontal profession. At the time, they were viewed as being radical, unproven, and unlikely to work. Not to mention that they posed a significant threat to the income of periodontists. Today, however, his research is widely accepted and praised. So much so, that consumer products companies routinely sell toothpaste containing hydrogen peroxide and baking soda.

Conventional treatment for periodontitis often requires surgery, called flap surgery, that involves cutting the gums, generally on two sides of each quadrant of the mouth. The gums are then peeled back, away from the roots of the teeth. The periodontist can then access the roots of the teeth to clean them and to repair bone, if necessary. They can also apply anti-bacterial medication on the roots and under the gums. The gums are then put back in place, and are sutured together.

This procedure is painful during surgery and for days later. The gums are very sensitive tissues and cutting them is quite painful, even with anesthesia. The procedure is generally done under local anesthesia in the periodontist's office. The gums are often discolored following the procedure, sometimes permanently. Often, the procedure needs to be repeated because the disease continues to progress.

Dr. Keyes identified the anaerobic bacteria that populate the gums, especially underneath them. He determined that hydrogen peroxide and baking soda were compounds that were hostile to these bacteria. He recommended a multi-week treatment process that could be done by dentists, with no need for periodontists. In the Keyes treatment, the teeth are scaled and cleaned free of tartar, an antibacterial solution is injected under the gum line, and the patient is required to daily irrigate the mouth with a water flosser and a solution of warm water, hydrogen peroxide and baking soda. No gum surgery is required or done.

Samples are taken from under the gums with cotton swabs, and then viewed under a microscope. The microscope is connected to a television monitor, so the patient can see for themselves the active community of bacteria living under their gums. This would often be recorded on a videotape as a history of the progress the patient was making. (DVDs came later). This visual demonstration was intended to motivate the patient to adhere to the home water flossing regimen because they could easily see for themselves the significant progress being made week by week — there would be dramatically fewer bacteria on the TV monitor at each successive visit to the dentist.

I tracked down a dentist who had been trained in the Keyes treatment methodology, and I religiously adhered to the home hygiene regimen of water flossing daily with warm water, hydrogen peroxide and baking soda. Within 90 days, my mouth had transformed dramatically. The pockets in my gums that cradled teeth had shrunk significantly. I no longer had bleeding gums. My periodontal disease was gone. My teeth were saved and my gums were healthy.[1]

At that time, I was vegetarian, but not vegan. That came later. But there is no question that my later conversion to a whole plant food lifestyle eliminated or reduced inflammation in my mouth and gums.

There is a well-known aphorism that speaks to this: "Don't look a gift horse in the mouth." I had wondered about the origin of this saying and found that it is rooted in health. For many centuries, when people bought and sold horses (or other livestock) they would examine the condition of its mouth. That is because the condition of an animal's mouth is a useful indicator of its general health. If the mouth is in poor condition, it indicates the animal has health issues, not only in its mouth but elsewhere in its body. This makes sense because if inflammation is present in the mouth it is likely present elsewhere in the body. So, if a horse had an unhealthy mouth, it was not a good buy. But if it was a free gift, don't bother looking at its mouth.

Since the time I used the Keyes technique to take care of my mouth, my gums are a healthy pink, my teeth are white and clean, and I have not lost a single tooth since that fateful day when I was 30 and I was told my teeth would fall out in my 60s. How vividly I remember the dentist telling me then that I had the mouth of someone twice my age. I am now 71 years of age. When I go to the dentist these days to have my teeth cleaned, the dentist is always amazed to see my teeth and gums. He tells me I have the mouth of someone half my age!

---

[1] Years later, when visiting Dr. Esselstyn and his wife, Ann, at their home in Cleveland, I was introduced to a good friend of theirs named Chuck Weller. At dinner, he complained about his periodontal disease, so I told him my story. Chuck immediately adopted the Keyes methodology and was amazed at the rapid improvement in his gums. He asked that I write the story for this book. Here it is, Chuck, for you and everyone else!

THE BENEFITS GO ON AND ON AND ON ...

Clearly, the benefits of a whole plant food lifestyle are numerous and have an impact throughout the body.

Now, when people tell me or my wife that we look decades younger than our age, I am not surprised. There is research that suggests a plant-based diet might slow the aging process in a number of ways, including by better preserving the protein-based telomere caps at the end of DNA strands, thus promoting healthier cell division. For centuries, humanity has been searching for the ever-elusive fountain of youth. It is none other than a WFPB lifestyle!

Now, when I hear male friends complaining about having to get up 2, 3 or more times a night to urinate because of an inflamed prostate, I empathize with them. But I am also very happy to not have to get up at all during the night to urinate, even at age 71. My prostate is not inflamed. A whole night's uninterrupted sleep is a wonderful thing!

Now, when I go to the ophthalmologist for my annual checkup and he is surprised that at age 71 I do not need reading glasses or have other vision issues, I thank my WFPB lifestyle for its never-ending benefits.

All these amazing benefits are available to everyone, without exception. ¬I tell people to try it for just 90 days. No matter how strongly someone objects, saying they could never give up meat or cheese, I say anyone can do it for 90 days.

Try it. What have you got to lose except suffering?

It is never too late to start feeling better.

Dan Purjes

HOPE
BY SCOTT STOLL, M.D.

**"May your choices reflect your hopes, not your fears"
– Nelson Mandela**

Hope is a very powerful and essential component of change. Throughout history a fresh infusion of hope instantaneously shifts the tide of the hardest-fought battle and empowers weakened survivors with renewed strength. Hope is the bridge that connects knowledge and inspiration to real life application. Our digital era places the highest value on information; it mistakenly believes that knowledge is all that we need to solve our problems. And, if we are still struggling, we just need more information or new knowledge to solve the problem.

In the case of chronic lifestyle diseases, the most comprehensive knowledge without hope and motivation is akin to an advanced Space X rocket with empty fuel tanks. It sits on the launch pad, gleaming in the sun, but doesn't have the energy to break free from gravity and fulfill its mission. This is where hope and motivation enter into the equation. Hope is the rocket fuel that propels knowledge off the launch pad, giving purpose and direction. Ignition is the moment someone visualizes a brighter future and believes that it is actually attainable. Then, hope motivates or fuels the right choices that lead to a brighter, healthier future.

"Wish upon a star."

When we were children, many of us learned the childhood song, "When you wish upon a star…your dreams come true," or the poem, "Star light, star bright, first star I see tonight, I wish I may, I wish I might, have this wish, I wish tonight ."

As adults we continue to "wish" for a better future, brighter circumstances or healthier life. But wishes are powerless. They passively depend on some outside force that magically brings the dream into reality.

Hope is very different. It is first conceived when we encounter someone like us who has overcome similar challenges, or when we discover a person who has solutions and resources that can help. Hope sparks something inside of us that says, "If they can do it, so can I." When that seed of hope takes root, people discover untapped internal reserves of strength and motivation that empower them to overcome obstacles and achieve lasting success.

The stories of transformed lives in this book inspire all of us to recognize new possibilities where hope and the science of nutrition unite. They are regular people who, like billions around the world, were struggling under the burden of a chronic disease until they discovered the hope-filled scientific pathway that led them to a brand new life of health and vitality. Day by day, they applied the science, one meal at a time. Within months, their lives were changed forever.

THE SCIENCE OF HOPE

What is hope and why is it important? It is a common word in our everyday conversations including comments like, "I hope it doesn't rain," "I hope I get a raise," and "I hope you feel better."

Authentic hope is more than passing comments or well wishes. It actually turns on the brain's pathways of success. Modern technology has allowed us to peer past the cranium into the mysterious inner workings of the brain and uncover some of the secrets of hope that have fueled courageous acts throughout history. Utilizing functional MRI techniques, measuring the blood flow and activity of different sections of the brain, researchers learned that when someone experiences hope it activates areas of the brain that are involved in long-term strategic planning and organization. Isn't that amazing? Hope turns on the areas of your brain that are necessary to achieve a goal or vision for a better future.

The bottom line is hope-filled people are able to visualize a brighter future, develop an achievable plan to get there, and immediately start taking positive, proactive steps in the right direction. Researchers also discovered that hope produces greater creativity, flexibility, and proactive risk-taking behavior to achieve the desired goal. We are more likely to step out and take a risk when we have hope!

Not surprisingly, hope-filled people naturally create new solutions and more easily change old habits to achieve their goals. Genuine hope launches an intense shift in brain activity that gives birth to a sincere belief that things can change, and it inspires decisive action. Scientific knowledge can only identify and recommend the correct steps that lead to consistent outcomes, but knowledge infused with hope creates an unstoppable force.

If hope is critical to long term success, then we all need to understand what inspires hope and where we can find more of it.

THE POWER OF STORY

Our brains have been hard-wired for stories. For thousands of years, stories were the primary method to pass on knowledge, wisdom, history and tradition to the generations that followed. History lessons were taught around campfires or fireplaces by parents and elders who instructed their children and prepared them for the future. Enchanting tales of heroes inspired bright-eyed children with wonder and hope as they believed that more is possible and that they, too, like their hero, could change the world. The oral stories became vivid memories in their mind's eye that would be frequently replayed and retold.

This powerful and effective transfer of knowledge and hope from one generation to the next is not merely a coincidence. In fact, we are similar to our ancestors in that our modern brains are still wired to respond to the empowering narrative of a story. A well-told story is something we all love. Whether it is in a book, on a movie screen, or around a campfire, we all settle in with great anticipation to hear or watch the story unfold. Years after we encounter a really good story, it lingers in our memory, evoking similar thoughts and emotions to the first day we experienced the story.

Science discovered that stories activate more than just our imagination. For example, when we learn new facts only two areas of our brain are activated. A well-spun story, however, fires up at least six regions of the brain at the same time, including the emotional memory centers and the brain's key reward centers. The emotional experience of a story releases chemicals in the brain, dopamine and oxytocin, that improve long-term memory and the ability to recall events with greater accuracy.

In fact, the research shows that a good story increases your capacity to remember information by at least seven times. This is evident in our own lives when we recall a memory of a favorite birthday, a vacation or a beautiful holiday. The memory instantly springs to life in ultrahigh definition. You can visualize the day in vivid color, smell the food cooking, hear the laughter, and see the smiling faces. We relive the event almost as if it was happening again and experience some of the same emotions.

Similarly, inspiring stories cause the brain cells, called neurons, to begin to fire together in unison, much like the beating of the heart. When neurons fire together, they also begin to wire together. Researchers call this neural coupling. Essentially, neurons begin to grow connections or bridges that connect to their neighbors and form a neural network that helps transfer and write the details of the story into long term memory. These newly "wired" connections help the reader or listener personalize the story with their own ideas, memories and experiences; essentially reliving the story through their own eyes. The author's story quickly becomes our own story, and the lessons they learned enlighten our own understanding and clarify the best pathway to success.

Stories also have the power to unite us in meaningful ways that cultivate community and offer support. Through a process called mirroring, readers or listeners of a story automatically begin to synchronize their brain activity with each other and with the storyteller. It is why we love to gather together as a group around a campfire, a dinner table or movie theater to enjoy the shared experience of a really good story; laughing, crying or holding our breath together as the story unfolds. People experience similar emotions, hopes or fears, and the story becomes a powerful shared experience that shapes group memories and beliefs. It also creates a unique space of shared history and connection when the story is retold.

We believe the stories in this book told by the people who lived them, and the shared experience by readers around the world will begin to reshape both individual and collective ideas about the possibilities of restoring health through a plant-powered plate. It is also our sincere desire that these stories will wire a new, powerful belief in your brain that their success is surely possible for you.

If stories are such a powerful tool, why haven't we integrated them into the delivery of healthcare? Data and information have become the currency of medical care and all too often, in the busyness of medical practice, long lists of information are given without a story or any thread to hold them together. The pieces of information are like individual leaves without branches or a trunk to give them context and support, and all too often they are blown away by the winds of busyness.

Interestingly, medical researchers have discovered that storytelling is significantly more effective to deliver medical guidance than fact-filled instructions. However, in most healthcare settings, the typical approach is to provide multi-page informational instructions. One study evaluated the treatment of high blood pressure and smoking cessation with instructions delivered as a story. Researchers discovered that the stories produced better and more statistically significant outcomes than the usual practice of providing informational instructions. A well-organized story can efficiently communicate complex ideas that are easily recalled and integrated into daily routines.

The science of nutrition can be very complex, but the story of a life transformed by lifestyle and nutrition is elegantly simple and inspiring. Stories engage the heart and the mind and at the same time and can make otherwise complex information easily understandable and memorable. We believe that each of the remarkable stories in this book will begin to assemble in your mind vital pieces of information about nutrition and lifestyle, and like a stained-glass window, become a new, beautiful and inspiring vision of health for your life.

Each of the hope-filled stories in this book represents the possibility and potential of restored health through a whole food plant-based lifestyle. This lifestyle is perhaps the greatest medicine because it has no side-effects, can be purchased without a prescription and doesn't require costly co-pays, deductibles or long wait times for a healthcare provider!

The best news is that you can start today and follow the "highlighted route" of the heroes in this book who have already succeeded.

Scott Stoll, M.D.

FROM HOPELESSNESS TO HEALTH
BY DAN PURJES

"Do not seek the truth; only cease to cherish opinions"
– Sosan, Third Patriarch of Zen

My co-author, Dr. Scott Stoll, began the previous chapter with a message of the importance of hope.

I will start my chapter with a message of hopelessness. The hopelessness that comes when someone reaches rock bottom. When their suffering is so intense and so awful that they are ready to abandon their cherished beliefs and opinions, ready to abandon their indelible illusions, their ingrained habits and defensive attitudes, and open to a new reality. A reality that is a radical departure from the way they have lived before, but that takes them to the new realm of health and vitality.

A wise man said: *"All that is true and beautiful and good, always exists as a paradox."*

The paradox here in this book is hopelessness and hope, both together. The hopelessness of being at rock bottom, with nowhere left to turn, and the hope that from rock bottom things can only get better. The hopelessness that says nothing seems to help, and the hope that, yes, there might still be a way. In many of the stories in this book, you will find this similar theme – hopelessness and hope that combine paradoxically and lead to a dramatically healthier life.

Every one of these stories is unique and different from the other stories, but they all involve hitting rock bottom and letting go of prejudicial, lifelong beliefs. Beliefs about what constitutes health, what is healthy to eat and what is not. Beliefs about the cause of chronic diseases or beliefs that their cause is unknown. Beliefs about how to deal with chronic diseases and the role of drugs. Beliefs that genes are destiny. Beliefs about what it takes to feel healthy, energetic and vibrant. Or even if that's possible.

It is only when they came to the end of their rope, the end of their hope, that the people who wrote these stories opened up and surrendered to change. They reached a place of hopelessness, where there was no longer any reason to hold on to cherished beliefs and illusions. They then opened to the realization that a whole plant food lifestyle held the answer to their suffering. And they began to hope again.

These cherished beliefs can be deadly: That diet has little to do with disease. That maximizing protein, especially animal protein, is the path to vitality, virility and health. That eating animal-based foods is important for good health; and that eating processed and packaged foods full of fats, sugars and salt is of no great concern. These beliefs are wrong and deadly.

What if you came to see that the standard America diet you consume every single day is deadly? That it is destroying your organs and your health, bit by bit? What if you came to realize the wisdom of Hippocrates when he said: "Let food be thy medicine"? Would that get you to change your diet?

Sosan, the Third Patriarch of Zen, said: *"Do not seek the truth; only cease to cherish opinions,"*

We all cling to beliefs and opinions. Most of the time, we don't even know why we believe what we do. We don't know where and how we came to believe what we believe. Many of our beliefs are from parents, family or friends; many came from media, marketing, and advertising, or from school, religion or jobs.

A professor of philosophy hiked up a hill to visit the Zen master, Nansen. He knocked and entered Nansen's house, sat down in a chair and asked, "What is truth?"

Nansen said, "Truth can wait. You're tired from hiking. Let me make you a cup of tea."

Nansen made the tea and began pouring it into the professor's cup. Until then, everything appeared normal. A tired man enters Nansen's house, and Nansen pours tea in a cup for refreshment. But then a strange thing occurred. The cup was full and Nansen kept pouring tea. The cup overflowed onto the saucer, yet Nansen continued to pour, and the tea overflowed onto the floor of Nansen's house.

"Stop!" yelled the professor. "Can't you see the cup is full? The tea is all over the floor!"

"Just so," said Zen Master Nansen. "Your mind is full of philosophy and opinions. How can truth enter?"

"You can see how the tea covers the floor," continued Nansen. "Now see how your beliefs and opinions cover your mind."

False beliefs and illusions in the world of health abound. *"Milk builds strong bones,"* or *"Meat is the best source of protein,"* or *"Carbs cause diabetes."* What if the opposite of those beliefs were true?

Beliefs that we are fat or sick because of our genes or our abnormal glands, so there's not much we can do about it. What if that were false much of the time?

Beliefs that chronic diseases cannot be reversed and the only option is to treat them with drugs or surgery. What if that was shown to be false again and again?

When the drugs fail or the surgeries are of no avail, despair sets in. When drugs lead to more drugs, when surgeries lead to more surgeries, and suffering continues unabated, hopelessness sets in. When we hit rock bottom, where hopelessness is overwhelming, we may finally let go of our cherished beliefs and illusions. And then the truth can enter. Change can begin. Healing can start. Hope returns.

"The unexamined life is not worth living," said Socrates.

When we are ready to give up these false, unfounded, unexamined beliefs, we can let new realizations enter our lives. When we stop clinging to cherished beliefs like, *"I could never give up meat,"* or *"I can't live without cheese,"* or *"I have a wicked sweet tooth,"* or *"It's because of my genes,"* then change can really begin. And the mastery of our own health can start.

Darkness is the absence of light. Truth is the absence of illusion.

When hopelessness leads to the abandonment of illusion, truth is revealed. Change can then come about and health begins.

That point of hopelessness in the stories in this book, was the point where change began. When those who suffered, surrendered their cherished illusions and opened up to a new reality, things got dramatically better. None of these people thought the food they ate was the cause of their misery. But when they discovered the truth and realized what a whole food, plant-based lifestyle could do for them, they converted. When they learned to distinguish between healthy food and unhealthy food, they changed what they ate.

In these stories, in the original authentic voice of these people, you will read how they reversed numerous diseases: Heart disease, cancer, diabetes, obesity, depression, lupus, rheumatoid arthritis, multiple sclerosis, and many other diseases. These people did what few people do today: reverse chronic disease without drugs or surgeries.

Most doctors do not believe that's possible. Some doctors, however, know it is true. The ones who know have lived it or have seen their patients live it, know it is true.

In this book there are stories by several doctors who themselves suffered from debilitating chronic diseases, who followed standard care practice, and went down the road of pharmaceuticals and medical procedures. They suffered horribly from side effects and pain. Only when they hit rock bottom, did they abandon the illusion that drugs were the answer and that diet had nothing to do with disease.

They learned about the healing benefits of whole plant foods. They converted to a whole plant food diet, and their diseases reversed and went into remission or disappeared completely. They learned to read ingredient labels, to avoid not only animal-based foods but packaged and refined foods full of sugars, fats, and salt. They learned about other healthy lifestyle factors such as exercising, sleeping and reducing stress. They adopted lifestyle factors wholeheartedly and healed their bodies.

These physicians reversed all kinds of chronic diseases in their own bodies – cardiovascular disease, hypertension, multiple sclerosis, lupus, rheumatoid arthritis, obesity, diabetes and other diseases.

People are sometimes surprised to hear that their physicians get sick, too. Don't they know better? No, they don't. They don't learn about nutrition in medical school or in residency or fellowship. Nutrition for the most part is not part of medical training.

One physician came down with multiple sclerosis (MS) at age 28. She had horrible adverse reactions to the medications she was told to take. She was told by her neurologist that if she did not take these terrible medications, she would likely wind up in a wheelchair by the time she was 50. It never occurred to her that food had anything to do with MS until she stumbled on a research article that mentioned the benefits of blueberries for MS patients. Blueberries? What does food have to do with MS, she wondered? As she pursued the connection of food to MS in several research articles, she realized food had enormous impact on MS and other autoimmune diseases. She converted to a whole plant food diet. Her neurologist dismissed that this would be of any help. But in her early 50s, when according to her neurologist she was destined to be in a wheelchair, she ran a 26-mile marathon.

In most instances the conversion to a whole food, plant-based diet was sudden and total. While some transition on a gradual basis, this can be difficult because it is harder to give up the sugar, processed food, and animal foods to which we are addicted. It is often easier and more effective to switch completely overnight. It was for me.

People are surprised to learn that animal foods are actually habit-forming. Animal based foods are frequently served with sauces and condiments that are loaded with sugar, fat and salt, all of which cause cravings. Dairy and dairy products like cheese are actually addictive. What would a cheeseburger taste like with no plant foods in the bun – no tomato, lettuce, pickles, or ketchup? Not even the bun! We humans have taste buds that are sensitized for plant foods, not for animal flesh.

"Where do you get your protein?"

This is a question that every plant-based person gets from many meat-eating people. It shows how pervasive illusions can be. There is only one source of protein on the planet -- plants!

All animals obtain protein by either eating plants or eating animals that eat plants. People are surprised to learn that animal foods are actually not the original source of protein. The protein in meat, poultry and fish all originate in plants, so eating animal foods provides a secondary, indirect source of protein, while eating plant foods provides a primary, direct source of protein. The protein in steak got there from the grass the cow ate.

People are also often surprised to realize, when it's pointed out to them, that the strongest land animals on the planet – elephants and gorillas – eat only plant food.

"Strong like a bull," is a popular saying. Bulls eat only plants.

Many people believe that humans are carnivorous. That's a false belief. When was the last time you salivated over road kill? If you were truly carnivorous, you would do so all the time, just like all carnivorous animals. In fact, if you were truly carnivorous, you wouldn't leave the roadkill there for other animals to grab. You'd stick your face in it and munch away, the way a cheetah, leopard or crow would do. (If that sounds disgusting to you, why would you think you are a carnivorous animal?)

People are surprised to learn that dairy is actually addictive. The addiction to dairy is similar to that of narcotics, but milder. The primary protein in milk is casein. When casein is digested, a byproduct called casomorphin is produced. It works on the brain just like morphine or opium, but more mildly. Scientists believe nature intended for casomorphin to promote pleasurable feeling and bonding between the newborn and its mother while nursing, and to encourage the newborn to consume mother's milk.

Of course, calves grow to be much larger than babies, so there is lots more casein in cow's milk, resulting in lots more casomorphins than nature intended for human beings – 10 or 15 times more by some estimates. And consider that it takes 10 pounds of milk to make 1 pound of cheese, and that means cheese can have 150 times the casomorphin levels intended by nature for human consumption. That explains the addictive hold cheese has on so many people. That also explains why the consumption of cheese increased 25-fold in the 20th century, and why the dairy industry is one of the largest food industries in the world.

Think about this: What mammalian species feeds milk to its young after they have been weaned and are eating solid food? None, except humans. What mammalian species feeds the milk of another species to its young? None, except humans.

This is but one example of an animal food that is not natural for humans to consume and which wreaks havoc on our bodies. Milk and cheese are major contributors to cardiovascular disease and cancer. They have been traced to many autoimmune diseases such as diabetes, lupus, rheumatoid arthritis and other chronic diseases. There is even some evidence connecting dairy to autism. Americans consume more dairy than ever before. Is it any wonder the incidence of these diseases is exploding?

Dairy marketing has persuaded people that milk is important for strong bones, but just the opposite is true. Cow's milk actually weakens bones and joints. Dairy digestion leads to an increased acidic level in the body. Calcium, an alkaline, is then leached from the bones to counteract the acidic condition. To see this clearly, note that the largest dairy consuming countries in the world per person are in North America and Western Europe, yet these are the very regions with the highest rates of bone fractures and joint replacements.

The countries with the lowest dairy consumption are in Southeast Asia, and they have the lowest rates of fractures and joint replacements, despite small-boned populations. If milk really "builds strong bones," just the opposite would be true.

"I have the fat gene, so I can't help being overweight."

It's astounding how many people believe genes are destiny. Not only do many people believe their health problems are attributable to genes, but their doctors believe it, too. We now know that genes account for only about 10% - 20% of health issues, yet most people and their physicians still harbor the illusion that genes are destiny.

The physician who got MS was told that genes were the probable cause, even though no one in her family had the disease. But genes are the explanation physicians often resort to when they don't know the cause of a disease, which is much of the time. She found it difficult to accept that genes were the cause of her MS, so she researched the medical literature on monozygotic (identical) twins and MS. Since identical twins have identical DNA, if one twin had MS, the odds of their twin sibling having MS should be 100%. But it turned out in scientific studies that the probability was only 14% - 30%.

If fat genes are to blame for obesity, why were there no obese people in the survivors of Holocaust concentration camps? They were all thin as skeletons.

There is a new medical science gathering lots of attention called epigenetics. This is the study of what activates genes. What turns them on. Genes are like a light switch. Having a switch does not mean the light is on. Genes are activated by environmental factors such as diet, exercise, stress, sleep, pollution, radiation and other factors. The most important of these much of the time is diet.

Animal based diets harm human health in many ways. Animal farming is destroying the planet. The greenhouse gasses generated by the raising of animals for food is greater than that produced by the entire transportation sector -- all cars, trucks, planes, trains, and ships. Vast areas of tropical forests, the "lungs of our planet," are being razed to provide grazing land for cattle. Enormous quantities of water go to raise animals for food — 4,000 gallons of water go to make just one hamburger. We face relentless drought partly because of animal farming.

All these problems can be easily remedied by conversion to a whole plant food lifestyle. All of humanity needs to do this, but it begins with each one of us individually. It has to begin with each one of us, individually. Each one of us can save humanity, can save the planet, can save the climate, can save water, and can save ourselves.

Health improvement begins almost immediately after converting to a whole, plant food lifestyle. Within a few days there are noticeable changes, and within weeks there's reversal of disease. Don't take our word for it. Try it for 30 or 60 days and see how you feel. There's nothing to buy except healthy, whole plant food. There's nothing to lose except excess weight, constipation and disease. Eat as much as you want, as long as what you eat is whole plant food. You'll be amazed at how quickly you lose weight and feel better, and how much energy and vitality you have.

Take control of your health. Take control of your happiness. Take control of your life.

Read the stories. The stories by people who had lost hope and found health again.

People who found hope again.

Dan Purjes

THE POWER OF A PLANT-BASED PLATE
BY DR. STOLL

"I did then, what I knew how to do. But now that I know better, I do better." Maya Angelou

Most of us have grown up in a world where processed foods and fast foods are the norm. Soda and sugary cereals for breakfast, donuts and coffee-with cream and sugar of course- at breaktime, candy bars and bagels in the afternoon and a fast-food meal on the way home. Without a second thought, we eat the way we were raised and programmed by our culture.

The industrialized food system filled with ultra-processed and convenience foods has coded our subconscious with automatic responses and habits that drive daily food choices. Until one day you wake up, press pause and begin asking the right questions: Why am I eating this and where did it come from? How was my food produced and what's in it anyway? What does my body need to really thrive? How do my food choices impact my wellbeing today and my disease risk and quality of life tomorrow? Is the sacrifice of my health and vitality worth the short term pleasure of processed and fast food? What is the true long term cost of "convenience" and cheap food? Is there a better way to eat that can prevent and reverse common diseases, and restore my health and vitality?

If you have never stopped to ask yourself these questions, please take a minute to re-read the above questions and answer them honestly.

The global pandemic of chronic, lifestyle disease is not caused by some unknown threat that will take science decades to unravel and develop a treatment. It is caused by the industrialized lifestyle and diet. Today, diet-related diseases like type 2 diabetes, high blood pressure and heart disease, impact more than 2 billion people worldwide. And according to numerous large studies, an unhealthy diet is the number one cause of death and disability in the United States.

It has been said that the truth can set you free, and a validated scientific truth is that the food you choose to eat every day is one of the most powerful forces on the planet to either heal or harm. The right choices can prevent, suspend and even reverse most common lifestyle related diseases like heart disease and type 2 diabetes, dramatically improve your immune system, protect you from infections, improve your mood and memory, and enhance your life. And you won't have to sacrifice taste in the process.

Truthfully, the "cure" is one of the most exciting dietary lifestyles that includes full plates and stomachs, abundant delectable food choices, normal body weight, reversal of many of the most common diseases like high blood pressure, type 2 diabetes, and irritable bowel syndrome, more energy, less pain, more mental clarity and hope for a brighter future. It is backed up by thousands of research studies and millions of people around the world that have stories of life transformation and disease reversal. It is not patented, nor does it require expensive prepared meals or supplements. The solution is a full plate of delicious whole plant-based foods that delight the taste buds and nourish the body with health promoting nutrients, which prevent and reverse disease.

DEFINING THE PROBLEM

In a 2017 Journal of the American Medical Association (JAMA) study, lead author Renata Micha PhD, RD said, "Our findings showed that the increased intake of certain foods and not enough of others was associated with nearly half of all deaths in the US due to heart disease, stroke, and diabetes."

Essentially, one out of every two deaths in the US could be prevented by the right diet. It also holds true for the global population. According to the Lancet Global Burden of Disease Study, 11 million deaths per year are linked to dietary risk factors. Metabolic lifestyle-related is increasing 1.5% per year. This shouldn't trigger fear because we know the solution and it is an immense opportunity to save lives and restore quality of life for people who are struggling under the burden of dietary related diseases.

Now, you may be asking yourself, "What types of food referenced in the JAMA study are the cause of premature death and disability and which foods are most important for disease prevention?"

Around the world today, the majority of people obtain more than 89% of their calories from processed food and industrialized animal products. Less than 11% of their calories are supplied by plants, and half of this category includes ketchup, French fries, and juice. Simply put, people are overfed, with too many calories from processed food and animal products, and yet immensely undernourished with minimal nutrients from plants. In fact, the Imperial College of London in 2017 recommended that maximum protection from disease could be obtained from 10 servings of fruits and vegetables per day.

Is public education enough to inspire change? The 5-a-Day campaign was launched more than 15 years ago to educate the public on the importance of eating 5 servings of vegetables and fruits per day. Follow-up research to determine the success of the program, revealed that 90% of people are aware of the US recommendation, and yet only 34% of people eat 2 or more servings per day. People are generally aware of the fact that they need to eat more plants but have not made changes to their daily habits.

WHY?

There are many potential reasons for this gap between knowledge and real life application. For example, educational campaigns have efficiently communicated to people "what to do" but have not inspired people with a compelling "why" to make the changes. Better numbers aren't inspiring. Lower blood pressure or reduced cholesterol are not very motivating, but spending time with grandchildren or achieving a life-long dream are empowering "why's" that help fuel change. Even a lower body weight may not be that inspiring unless it is connected to a meaningful "why" like a wedding, beach vacation, or class reunion.

You see, knowledge is not the only ingredient needed for change. In the 21st century digital era we have mistakenly come to believe that more knowledge is the answer to everything, but in the case of a lifestyle change it is only one component. The recipe for success also includes inspiration, hope, support, community, resources, training, persistence, and love. With these ingredients, and allowed to bake for 6 months, this recipe is a guaranteed winner. Watch for each of these elements in the stories in this book and make a note on how you can add them to your life.

100 BITES PER DAY

Did you know that in your lifetime you will eat approximately 87,000 meals, 140,000 pounds of food and at least 50 million calories? The positive or negative effect of all of this food really adds up quickly, and it is easy to see that trying to balance 50 million calories to control weight over a lifetime is nearly impossible. But your health is far more than balanced calories and weight management.

The 100 bites of food that enters your body every day are not just protein, fat and carbohydrates with a total daily calorie number that needs to be balanced by sweating it out on a treadmill. Every bite that we put into our mouths has a positive or negative impact on our cells within hours. Food is either packed with supportive nutrients that reduce inflammation, rebuild cells and maintain a disease resistant body, or loaded with substances that ignite inflammation, injure cells, deplete resources, suppress the immune system, steal vitality, energy, and clarity, and leave behind disease, pain and suffering.

Food is never neutral; it either supports and nourishes, or it inflames and injures. Bite by bite either the injury level increases until the disease debt bankrupts health or health accrues yielding an inheritance of vitality, energy, and resilience. As you begin to eat more positive than negative calories, your body will initiate healing; and as you add more whole plant foods every day, the healing cycle accelerates.

Food is far more complex than simply balancing calories or manipulating protein, fat or carbohydrates. This is where the diet industry has it all wrong. Decades of dietary research has shown on average that only 15% of people succeed in keeping off twenty pounds for 5 years. The other 85% who unsuccessfully tried dieting often feel stuck, frustrated, powerless, guilty and even hopeless. The dieting industry has failed millions of people because **dieting simply doesn't work**. Vibrant enduring health and sensible weight management will never be found in a short-term fad diet, secret new formula or breakthrough supplement. Instead, true health and normal weight are found on a beautiful whole food, plant based plate and through lifestyle choices.

If you have struggled with dieting in your past, we want to tell you that it is not your fault, and encourage you right now to release any guilt, shame or self-condemnation associated with dieting. The diet and healthcare industries in general did not provide you with the right information and the critical support that you needed to make a lasting change. We want you to know that we believe in you and support you, as do all of the people who shared their stories in this book. And we know that if you connect with some of the great communities and resources highlighted in this book and apply the basic principles consistently, every day trying to "do better" than yesterday, you will succeed.

FOOD FOR LIFE

A well planned, whole food, plant-based lifestyle, on the other hand, gets it right on every level. It contains all of the protein, fat, and carbohydrates necessary to build a healthy body. Plants are the richest sources of fiber and micronutrients such as vitamins, minerals, antioxidants and phytochemicals. Bite by bite the nutrients work together like a symphony in your body to reduce inflammation, promote healing, support your immune system, normalize blood sugars and in many cases reverse diseases like heart disease, high blood pressure and type 2 diabetes. True lasting success is always found in consistent daily lifestyle choices of delicious whole food plant powered meals, regular activity, 7-8 hours of sleep, healthy community and releasing stress.

How can we know that a plant-based diet is the healthiest way to eat?

First, we start with a big picture view, looking at the longest lived and the healthiest groups of people from around the world. They in areas called blue zones. These unique regions include the cities or islands of Ikaria, Greece; Loma Linda, California; Okinawa, Japan; Sardinia, Italy; and Nicoya, Costa Rica. Researchers studying these populations discovered that they shared many similar health promoting diets and lifestyle practices. For example, they generally consumed a 95% plant-based diet that included one cup of beans or lentils each day, maintained daily physical activity and lived in supportive communities. As a result, these groups of people were found to have almost non-existent levels of chronic diseases, like heart disease, high blood pressure, and type 2 diabetes. They reach age 100 at rates ten times more than the US population, live healthy and productive lives and don't spend their time waiting in a doctor's office or pharmacy line.

Alternatively, America and the majority of the westernized world today are red zones. According to the U.S. Department of Agriculture 57% of our calories are from processed and fast foods, 32% from animal based foods and only 11% from plants. The result is that the majority of the daily calories for most people are filled with inflammatory ingredients – sugars, saturated fat, oils, preservatives, refined flour, and preservatives that injure the body. Additionally, the majority of people are inactive, sleep too little, stress too much and don't have supportive communities. The result: unprecedented levels of chronic disease, runaway healthcare costs and lost time in sick beds, hospitals, doctor's offices and pharmacies.

The COVID-19 pandemic spotlighted the risks of an unhealthy lifestyle. Obesity is associated with a 46% higher risk of infection, 74% greater risk for ICU admission and 48% higher rate of death. Those with the worst lifestyle scores were 300% more likely to get a COVID-19 infection. The evidence points to an unhealthy lifestyle as the greatest risk factor for a severe or fatal case of COVID-19. Approximately 80% of the COVID-19 related deaths are in people over age 65 and research has found that 85% of the people in this group have at least one lifestyle related disease. Nearly two thirds of patients hospitalized for treatment of COVID-19 symptoms were obese or overweight, and 70% had high blood pressure.

Lifestyle related diseases like heart disease, diabetes, lung disease and immune-compromised conditions all resulted in a greater likelihood of hospitalization and or death. The choices we make matter in more ways than we might imagine and are magnified by events like the COVID-19 pandemic. Therefore, a healthy lifestyle and whole food plant-based diet may be one of the most important, effective and protective public healthcare interventions against infectious pandemics like COVID-19. Based on these statistics, it is imperative that we rapidly move toward a nutrient rich diet for the health of our families and nations.

Plant-based diets are known to fortify and boost the immune system. What better defense against COVID-19 can there be than a strong immune system?

RESTORATION

Restored health and disease reversal are built on the foundation of a whole food plant based plate. The good news is that every delicious bite of a whole food plant-based meal is packed with all of the nutrients and fiber that supports healing and normal function. **Remember this truth: your body's natural state is health, not disease.** And when you feed your body the right food and create a restorative environment through sleep, exercise, and stress reduction, it will begin to heal and stabilize disrupted systems immediately. In a very short period of time the symptoms of disease, like high blood pressure, elevated blood sugars, angina, or chest pain can begin to dissipate and may even disappear. Why? Because you are providing your body with the time, resources and opportunity to repair, regenerate, and heal.

Whole plant foods are the jump start your body needs and every bite contains:

- Fiber that feeds the bacteria in your microbiome (50 trillion bacteria that live in your gut) and in return it supports the health of your entire body. We get back far more than we put in! The fiber in plants feeds the beneficial strains of bacteria that stabilize blood sugars, reduce inflammation, heal the gut lining, strengthen the immune system, and improve brain function and mood. Fiber also helps to wash away excess cholesterol and estrogen. Sadly, only 4% of people today consume the recommended amount of fiber.

- Antioxidants and phytochemicals (the part of plants that give them color like the blue in blueberries or the orange in carrots) that heal DNA, reduce inflammation, protect against cancer, fight bacteria and viruses, build stronger bones, enhance the microbiome and improve blood flow to the heart and brain.

- Minerals that enhance cellular reactions in every part of the body. Whole unprocessed plants grown in organic soil are the richest source of minerals and phytochemicals.

- Vitamins that optimize enzyme function, improve metabolism, aid in the growth of ligaments, bone, and connective tissue, build red blood cells, and heal nerves, just to name a few of their many vital activities.

- And plenty of plant protein, healthy fats, and complex carbohydrates that provide all of the necessary energy and building blocks for a strong, energetic disease-free body.

Recent research has shown that fiber is critical to your health. Years ago, researchers didn't know about the microbiome (the 50 trillion bacteria that live in your intestinal system) and believed that fiber's only function was to aid digestion and avoid constipation. Today we know that the microbiome is incredibly complex and has many important jobs including; maintaining a healthy immune system, reducing inflammation throughout the body and in the colon, maintaining the health of gut lining, communicating with the brain, and stabilizing blood sugars, to name just a few of the microbiome's important functions. To accomplish this critical work, the microbiome needs lots of food, and fiber is its food! It is important to know that fiber is only available in plant foods. Processed and animal based foods do not contain fiber. And the good news is that when your plate is powered by plants, you don't ever need to worry about getting enough fiber!

CALORIE DENSITY: THE KEY TO HEALTHY WEIGHT

Dr. Barbara Roll and her team at Penn State University discovered that people who eat a diet of about 600 calories per pound of food will maintain a normal healthy body weight. In fact, according to their research you can eat all the food you want at 300 calories per pound and never gain a pound. Between 300-800 calories per pound, you can eat large portions and maintain a healthy body weight, depending slightly on your activity level. Foods with a calorie density of 800-1,800 per pound should be strictly limited as these can contribute to weight gain and limit weight loss. Additionally, the intake of foods over 1,800 calories per pound should be extremely limited to very small occasional servings as these foods can easily contribute to weight gain and obesity.

The 2007 report from the American Cancer Institute and the World Cancer Research Fund also recommended lowering the average calorie density of the American diet to 567 calories per pound to lower the risk of cancer. You can easily do this by following the above principles and the chart below of calorie density. These allow us to eat freely unrefined, unprocessed fruits, vegetables, starchy veggies, intact whole grains and legumes (with no added salt, sugar and fat/oil).

By now, I bet you can probably guess what types of foods are approximately 600 calories per pound or less. You're right! Whole plant foods. Take a look at this chart that was created from scientific data.

Calorie Density Chart

FOOD	CALORIES PER POUND
Vegetables	60-100
Fruit	100-425
Potatoes/Yams	300-600
Whole Grains	325-625
Lentils/Beans/Peas	500-700
Avocado	750
Dried Fruit	1000
Bread, Bagels, Muffins	900-1300
Animal Protein/Dairy/Ice Cream	1200
Cheese/Sugar/Soft Drinks	1600-1800
Fried Foods and Snacks	2000-2400
Chocolate	2500
Nuts and Seeds	2800
Butter	3500
Oil	4000

A diet of whole plant foods falls largely above the red line and provides all of the necessary nutrition without excess calories. Notice that there are a few whole plant-based foods below the red line, like avocados at 750 calories per pound, dried fruits 1000 and nuts and seeds 2800, and should only be consumed in small amounts occasionally. Processed plant foods can be much higher in caloric density and similar in calorie density to animal products at 1200 calories per pound. They should be minimized and only eaten rarely.

Did you happen to see the number of calories per pound for oil? At 4000 calories per pound, or 120 calories per tablespoon, oil is a highly calorie-dense processed food that leaves you feeling hungry. Yes, that also includes olive oil. The same olive oil that many people use to cook food and douse their salads and pasta. The majority of refined vegetable oils, but not olive oil, are high in Omega 6 fatty acids that can trigger inflammation. All oils are processed[1], calorie dense and ideally prepared for rapid storage as body fat. I often like to joke "lips to hips in 3 minutes!." Oil can sneak into your diet in many places, even in the delicious salad dressing on your healthy restaurant salad. The salad is a good choice, but the oily dressings are not. In fact, restaurants use on average 4-5 tablespoons (480-600 calories of dressing!) on a salad. So, to lose more weight or just maintain a healthy weight, lose the oil and use alternative dressings like a delicious balsamic or flavored vinegar instead.

FULL AND FULFILLED

A whole food, plant-based lifestyle will change your life. Unlike diets designed to starve and deprive the body of calories, a whole plant food lifestyle is about abundance, freedom, a vibrant life, fulfillment, and large delicious meals with a full plate- and stomach – all while maintaining a healthy weight.

A whole food plant-based diet effectively turns off hunger signals in at least three ways. First, as seen in the diagram below, the high volume of fiber in a whole food plant-based diet rapidly fills the stomach and activates the stretch receptors in the stomach wall. The receptors send a signal the hunger centers in the brain that the stomach is full and the hunger alarm can be turned off.

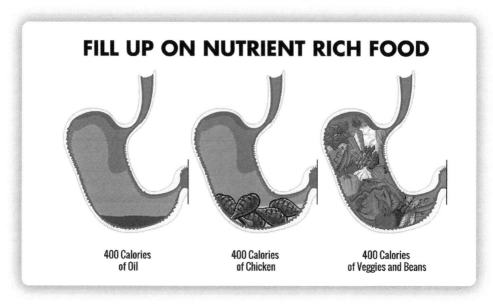

FILL UP ON NUTRIENT RICH FOOD

| 400 Calories of Oil | 400 Calories of Chicken | 400 Calories of Veggies and Beans |

Second[2], the nutrients in the plants, the phytochemicals that give plants their color, turn off the hunger signals in the area of the brain called the hypothalamus. Once the brain receives the message that the body has received enough nutrients it messages the hand to put down the fork and spoon.

Finally, plants rich in fiber and phytochemicals feed the bacteria that live in your digestive system. The bacteria feast on the fiber from the plants at breakfast lunch and dinner and just like any factory, produce waste or by-products. The by-products like short chain fatty acids are not waste, but a valuable resources for your health. One of their many contributions to a healthy body is the ability to turn off cravings and hunger and contribute to the satisfaction of feeling fulfilled at the end of a meal.

STARVING BODIES

It may seem strange, but when a person is overweight or obese, they are actually starving for nutrients and experience frequent hunger pangs. Hunger is the body's way of alerting the "user" to go and consume nutrient rich food to meet the need. When they seek to satisfy those hunger pangs, people tend to do so with the nutrient poor diet common to our culture that is filled with processed and refined foods, or with animal based products. This sets up a vicious cycle of hunger followed by unhealthy food choices with insufficient nutrient intake and excessive calories and within two to three hours the alarm bell of hunger sounds again. Combined with this cycle, cravings and emotional eating can also masquerade as hunger.

Additionally, unhealthy foods are high in processed sweeteners that only briefly quiet hunger and add empty, inflammatory calories. When the body realizes that it didn't receive the nutrients it needs and it is inflamed, it sounds the alarm bell of hunger, and another cycle of consuming processed and refined foods, and animal based products, begins. This vicious cycle will never end until nutrient rich food is eaten to provide the needed nourishment.

FLATTENING THE CURVE

Your body's natural state is health. I can't emphasize this point enough. Most diseases occur when outside influences like diet, stress, inactivity and toxins injure cells and deplete critical body resources. Bite after bite of unhealthy food, one stressful inactive day after another results in the accumulation of small cellular injuries much like a credit card debt accumulates, one swipe at a time. Your body diligently works to keep you going every day by making small withdrawals from its precious reserve accounts until one day they are depleted and your body faces a crisis.

Eventually, the cellular injury reaches a critical tipping point, much like a credit card debt that reaches the credit limit. This is the point when disease symptoms begin to manifest like the chest pain of heart disease, the elevated blood sugars and frequent urination of type 2 diabetes, or the joint pain and swelling of rheumatoid arthritis. The body is essentially overwhelmed by persistent and chronic cellular injury and reaches a state where systems begin to fail. Sometimes this failure can be life threatening.

The western diet and lifestyle are harmful. With every unhealthy bite and inactive, stress filled day, inflammation smolders and cell damage accumulates until the body hits the tipping point. Just before the body reaches its limit and is no longer able to function normally, warning signs begin to appear. These are early notifications that a lifestyle change is needed before the "check engine light" of disease appears on your dashboard. The early signs may include fatigue, pain, exhaustion, indigestion, inflammation, or constipation and typically precede a measurable, clinical diagnosis. If someone tries to silence the warning signals with medications that manage the symptoms, or caffeine to overcome fatigue, and food, alcohol, or substances to treat stress, they may be on their way to a major breakdown and new disease diagnosis. It is critically important to learn to listen to your body. When it is tired, get a good night's sleep, when it is hungry feed it food that nourishes and heals, when it is stressed breathe, release, and rest.

The good news is that if an unhealthy lifestyle causes the system failure, in the majority of cases, an intensive lifestyle intervention can turn back the clock and jump start the healing process and flatten the curve. Hippocrates said, "Healing is not just a matter of time, but also opportunity." A whole food, plant-based lifestyle provides both the time and opportunity to help the body reverse the harmful effects of the standard western diet and lifestyle.

An important note of clarification for the concept of disease reversal or remission, is this: Diseases are diagnosed based on a constellation of findings – symptoms, physical examination, lab work and other data like biopsies and imaging findings (MRI, CT, X-ray). As the body heals, these characteristic findings can also resolve. Essentially, the disease condition goes into remission with no further symptoms or measurable evidence of the disease condition. However, the susceptibility is still present and it remains silenced through healthy lifestyle choices. If someone returns to the same lifestyle that caused their disease, the disease condition and symptoms can return.

TYPE 2 DIABETES
Extensive research on plant-based diets for type 2 diabetes have shown:

- A whole food, plant-based lifestyle is the best prevention for type 2 diabetes and the surest way to reverse it.

- Significant improvements, and in many cases, normalization of hemoglobin A1c and blood glucose levels result from adopting a whole plant food lifestyle. In controlled trials, 74% of people on oral medications and 44% of people on insulin were able to discontinue medications in 4-12 weeks.

- Severe pain of diabetic peripheral neuropathy can be dramatically improved in 81% of patients in just 4-16 days.

- A whole plant food lifestyle leads to improved beta cell function in the pancreas with increased production of insulin.

- A whole plant food lifestyle leads to improved kidney function, wound healing, and reduced risk of blindness.

- A whole plant food lifestyle leads to lower cholesterol, risk of heart disease, stroke, and cancer for people living with diabetes.

The common belief is that consumption of carbohydrates causes type 2 diabetes. Refined carbohydrates like sugar and refined flour are not healthy and can contribute to insulin resistance. But it is the consumption of fats, oils, and excessive animal food products, combined with processed food, that really stokes the fires of inflammation and insulin resistance. People who reversed type 2 diabetes on a plant-based diet included many fresh whole fruits in that diet with blood glucose or A1c issues.

China provides a compelling case study. For centuries, white rice and plant based foods were a staple in Chinese diets. Until the 1980s, type 2 diabetes was rare in China. But in the mid 1980;s that began to change as newfound prosperity brought an abundance of processed food, fast food and animal food products to Chinese tables. Today, type 2 diabetes rates in China are similar to that of the US. In just 40 years, China went from very low rates of type 2 diabetes to one of the largest diabetes populations on the planet.

HEART DISEASE AND HIGH BLOOD PRESSURE

Numerous studies, including the Landmark Lifestyle Heart Trial, have shown that with a whole plant food diet:

- Heart disease can be halted, and in many cases reversed, and angina (non-emergency chest pain) can be resolved. The blood supply can be restored to damaged areas of the heart through a whole food, plant-based lifestyle, thus eliminating angina pain.

- Cholesterol is normalized.

- High blood pressure can be improved without medication, through a whole plant-based diet; medications are frequently reduced or discontinued in many cases beginning in just 1 week

- Increased exposure to antioxidants and phytochemicals lowers inflammation levels, protects the delicate cell lining of your arteries, called the endothelium, which helps provide critical elasticity to blood vessels, and optimizes blood flow to every part of your body.

- Significantly reduces the risk of stroke

- And, in some cases, an intensive lifestyle intervention can dramatically improve heart failure.

Additionally, a whole food plant-based lifestyle improves many common conditions including:

- Powerfully reduces inflammation and pain

- Calms and helps to heal IBS/IBD

- More effectively reduces weight than any other dietary lifestyle

- Improves, and in many cases, reverses autoimmune diseases like rheumatoid arthritis, lupus, multiple sclerosis, and chronic kidney disease

- Clears asthma

- Improves mood

- Diminishes allergies

- Ends constipation

- Resolves acne

- Halts PCOS

- Prevents dementia

- Reduces arthritic pain

- Improves renal impairment

- Significantly reduces the risk of colon and other cancers

- And many more.

All systems normal

To top it all off, a plate of delicious whole plant food normalizes the growth of blood vessels in your body to heal injured or damaged tissue and prevents the growth of abnormal blood vessels that supply cancer and fat cells. It also heals the intestinal cells, normalizes bowel movements, turns off key inflammation master switches, reduces inflammation in the brain and improves mood and feelings of well-being.

In fact, the growing body of research is discovering that a plant-based diet is good for every part of your body.

DO IT!

Congratulations on your decision to take control of your health destiny and future.

Remember that your body is the only vehicle you have to transport you through life – and there are no trade-ins after 50,000 miles! A strong healthy body provides you with abundant opportunities and adventures that are impossible with a failing body.

It is important to recognize that healthcare systems have limitations. They can't accomplish what you can when you decide to change what's on your plate two to three times per day. It begins with the "self-care" decisions that you will make today about what's on your plate, on your fingers and fork, and how much you will move and sleep and release stress. Your health future truly is in your hands.

8 SIMPLE STEPS FOR CHANGE

1. Find your empowering "why" for change. It should be a core motivation for your life or a passionate vision/dream for the future. Your "why" may include dreams for the future such as being with and loving a family, being with and loving your grandchildren, serving around the world, impacting your community, sharing your gift or completing a challenging event like a triathlon. What's yours?

2. Develop a basic game plan with a series of small goals that are easily achieved and regularly celebrated. These small, achievable steps are the key to changing habits. Set a goal that seems so small that your brain says, "That's it! I can do it easily!" Once you accomplish that goal, celebrate your success and set another small goal. Just like stepping stones, these successful small goals lead you to a full healthy lifestyle. For example, commit and convert to a whole food, plant-based diet for just 30 days. If you find that you feel much better, have more energy, fewer aches and discomfort, are more regular and sleep better, go another 30 days. And so forth. Before you know it, you will never look back!

3. Find a tribe—surround yourself with a support group of like-minded and motivated people. Research has taught us that every part of our lives, including finances and our microbiome, will become similar to our closest friends. Search out a supportive group, ideally in person, but an online community can also be a great resource for support and encouragement.

4. Start and progress toward a 100% whole food, plant-based dietary lifestyle: There is no more powerful influence on your health than your diet. Food is never neutral and will either support and strengthen your body or damage and erode your health. A simple action step might include purging your pantry and refrigerator of unhealthy, disease promoting, processed foods, or planning a weekly menu rich in vegetables and fruits, or stopping to pick up the ingredients for a green smoothie. Create an environment to thrive at home by placing healthy choices in prominent places that are easy to see and easier to access. Ideally, remove all of the potentially tempting, harmful foods

from your home. This will greatly improve your ability to succeed and will help you to build self-discipline over time without the constant pull of unhealthy food in your home.

5. Stress: If you were playing the card game of health, stress would be the wild card. Stress can quickly erode a healthy body and studies have linked it to many diseases such as cancer, heart disease, autoimmune diseases, immune suppression, high blood pressure, and stroke. Stress is a given in life, but the key is to learn how to minimize prolonged stress and cut loose unnecessary sources of stress. Perspective is a key to overcoming stress. Intentionally take some time to step back from the situation and place the stressor in the context of world events and your lifetime. Another simple action step that you can take is to stop and practice deep breathing. Slow, rhythmic breaths in through the nose, hold, and out through the mouth helps the body release the physical effects of stress and normalize blood flow and hormonal levels. Be mindful of your breathing as you take each breath. Pay attention to the breath coming in and then going out. Five deep breaths three times per day can dramatically lower your stress levels! Try it today.

6. Toxins: Tobacco, alcohol, and drugs destroy cells in the body and even low levels of toxins in our food and household products can trigger chronic inflammation. The largest contributor to free radical damage of the cells and DNA is tobacco. Regular participation in any of these activities will result in long-term damage to the body and the need for health care services. It is important to recognize the harmful effects of toxins and choose a toxin free life including removing toxic inputs from food and your home.

7. Activity: Every day we have a choice to move or sit. Our culture promotes sitting: sitting at a meal table, at your desk, in the car, on the couch. It is important to recognize that your body needs to move to be healthy. In fact, research has suggested that sitting in the 21st century is equivalent to smoking in the second half of the 20th century. Every day, look for simple opportunities to move more, such as taking the stairs whenever possible, walking, not sitting, when you are on the phone. (I am trying to stand while editing this book). Work on your posture when sitting or standing, and schedule time for movement and stretching five times per week. Make it fun to find something you really enjoy.

8. Celebrate Success: Self-care recognizes the emotional, relational, physical and financial rewards of good health. The money that might have been spent on copays, deductibles, procedures or the money lost sick days missed at work can be reallocated to celebrate a long-anticipated vacation, or a wonderful healthy meal catered into your home for friends and family, a shopping spree or simply saved for

another day. The celebration will help to solidify the tangible benefits of your decision and make any perceived sacrifices worthwhile. A healthy lifestyle opens wide the doors of opportunity; eat wisely, live peacefully, move frequently, breathe deeply, and appreciate the gift of your life.

Choose wisely, live richly.

Scott Stoll, M.D.

---

[1] Almost all oils, even plant-based oils, use petroleum solvents to extract oil from the plant. The only exception are cold-pressed oils such as cold-pressed, extra virgin olive oil. However, even that oil is extremely high in calories and has almost no nutrients.

THE COVID-19 PANDEMIC
BY SCOTT STOLL, M.D. AND DAN PURJES

At the time we started working on this book in 2019, the COVID-19 pandemic and the coronavirus that caused it, SARS-CoV-2, was unknown to the general public. Then in early 2020, it burst onto the scene and changed the world forever.

As of the publication of this book, the WHO estimates that hundreds of millions of people have been infected with this disease and many millions have died. Scientists raced to understand the virus, and through hundreds of clinical trials sought to develop new vaccines and effective treatments. To date, three vaccines in the US have been granted emergency use authorization by the US Food and Drug Administration, and two anti-viral treatments have been similarly been approved.

One of the pressing questions amongst researchers is, "Are there common characteristics in those who have moderate to severe cases or have died from COVID-19?" The answer is a resounding yes! The majority were overweight or obese, older than 60 and had a concurrent disease condition such as type 2 diabetes or high blood pressure. All these conditions indicate a weaker immune system. Current statistics have highlighted risks of more severe cases associated with lifestyle related diseases.

- People with type 2 diabetes are 3 times more likely to have severe symptoms

- Hypertension increases the risk of mortality by 3.5 times

- Patients with pulmonary disease are at higher risk of dying from COVID-19

- People who are obese are seven times more likely to have severe symptoms

- Long term complications, or long-haul COVID, are more likely in obese people

The trifecta for severe complications or death is men over age 60 with obesity and a chronic disease like type 2 diabetes or hypertension. At the core of many of these risk factors is inflammation and a weakened immune system. Conditions like obesity, type 2 diabetes, and the western diet, continually produce inflammation and suppress the immune system. Then, when the body is attacked by a virus like COVID-19, the immune system tries to jump into action but is too weak to respond correctly.

Normally, the body responds to a viral infection like COVID-19 with a controlled burst of inflammation to kill off the invading viral forces. But, in the case of severe COVID-19, the weakened and confused immune system responds with an excessive burst of inflammation, called a cytokine storm, that damages delicate, vital tissues like the blood vessel walls in the heart and lungs. A healthy diet supports a healthy immune system that can efficiently respond to infections. Numerous studies have documented the anti-inflammatory effect of a whole food plant based diet and its ability to build a strong immune system.

Antioxidants and phytochemicals are naturally occurring substances in plants that reduce inflammation. The microbiome, the community of trillions of bacteria in the human digestive tract, feeds on the fiber in plant foods and produces numerous health promoting by-products, called short chain fatty acids (SCFA). The SCFA's reduce inflammation locally in the gut and are transferred throughout the body to improve everything from insulin sensitivity to brain function.

In just weeks on a whole food plant-based diet, markers of inflammation, like C-Reactive Protein (CRP), are substantially reduced in people who were either overweight or obese. Those with the healthiest plant-based diets experience the greatest reduction in inflammation compared to those who consume a less healthy, more processed plant based diet.

Protein has been the focus of the diet industry for decades. However, we do not have a protein deficiency in our country, we have a crisis of fiber deficiency. Less than 4% of the population consumes the recommended amount of daily fiber. In fact, many scientists consider the daily recommendation of 20-25 grams to be too low. The question people should be asking is not, "How much protein am I getting today?", but rather, "How much fiber am I getting today?" Without sufficient fiber, the healthy bacteria in the gut that support the immune system, are replaced by bacteria that shift the body into an inflamed state and create an inefficient immune system.

Simply connecting the dots helps us to see the best pathway forward.

- Just about everyone, including the majority of researchers, would agree that the more fresh fruits and vegetables, and other whole plant foods, a person eats, the stronger their immune system.

- And just about everyone would also agree that the stronger a person's immune system, the more likely they are to resist the adverse effects of any disease, chronic or infectious, including COVID-19.

- Therefore, it is simple logic that a whole plant food diet is the best diet to protect against COVID-19, and unquestionably better than the standard American diet or an animal-based diet.

Does scientific research bear out that a whole food plant based diet protects you from COVID-19? New evidence suggests, YES, and the benefits may be very significant.

Thousands of front-line COVID-19 healthcare workers from six countries were followed for moderate to severe outcomes from a COVID-19 infection. Those who followed a plant based diet had three fold lower probability of a moderate to severe case; pescatarians (plants plus fish), had a two-fold lower probability; and those on a low carbohydrate, high protein diet (e.g. keto diet) had a significantly increased probability of a moderate to severe case. Similarly, poor sleep and high levels of burnout, were associated with greater odds of moderate to severe cases of COVID.

These are the first studies of their kind, but more research is underway and we predict that the evidence will continue to stack up in favor of a plant-based diet and healthy lifestyle. Your plant powered plate will help to protect you from COVID-19 and it will aid in the recovery if you contract the disease and battle its aftereffects.

Begin today by fortifying your defenses against COVID-19 with a transition to a whole food plant based diet and a healthy lifestyle.

Scott Stoll, M.D. and Dan Purjes

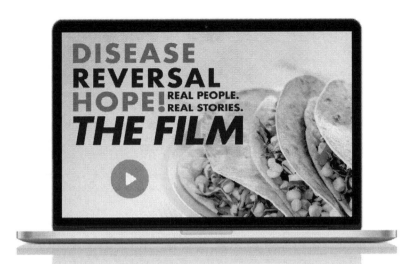

DISEASE REVERSAL HOPE: The Film is a full length documentary that brings to life many of the stories in the book, *DISEASE REVERSAL HOPE! Real People. Real Stories.* The filmmakers of, Eating You Alive, have filmed a new, full-length documentary of *Disease Reversal Hope!* The stories in the book come alive as the storytellers vividly describe their ordeal and journey to health.

Both the book and the film share stories of people who suffered from horrible chronic diseases, people who were told nothing could be done for them, people who hit rock bottom and stared at the abyss of a hopeless future. People who were told they only had months to live. These people found their way to a whole food, plant-based lifestyle that reversed their diseases and gave them a new, vibrant life. These are the people who tell their stories in *DISEASE REVERSAL HOPE: The Film.* In the documentary, new details are revealed and the gripping stories take on an added dimension.

The filmmakers of *Eating You Alive,* director and producer Paul David Kennamer, and their film crew and producer Merrilee Jacobs traveled the country in their RV bus, a mobile film studio, meeting, interviewing and filming people who contributed their stories to the book. The result is a powerful new rendition of the book. Dan Purjes, co-author of the book, was the Executive Producer of the film, as well as a co-producer.

Please tell your family and friends about the book and the film.
Help spread health.

The film is owned by the Purjes Foundation, as is the book. The Purjes Foundation is a non-profit charitable trust that supports health of body, mind, and soul, founded and privately funded by Dan and Edna Purjes (**www.PurjesFoundation.org**). The Purjes Foundation is paying all the costs incurred in connection with the production of the film and book. All proceeds, net of expenses, from the sale of the book and the film will go to charities that support plant-based nutrition. **The book and film can be purchased or rented at:**

DISEASEREVERSALHOPE.ORG OR ON AMAZON

EATING YOU ALIVE

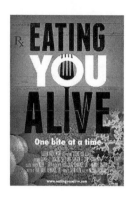

Eating You Alive is a gripping documentary film that shows how the lives of many different people were dramatically changed when converting to a whole plant food lifestyle. They were able to reverse horrible, and often fatal, chronic diseases. Heart disease, cancer, diabetes and numerous autoimmune diseases are all reversed, often in a relatively short period of time.

These people had horrendous prognoses, in many cases fatal, and agonizing symptoms and painful adverse side effects to prescribed drugs. Each of them reversed diseases. In some cases the reversal was so effective that even in the case of diseases predicted to be terminal, there was no longer any detectable disease in the body. These are people who were told by physicians that there was nothing more medicine could do for them, and that they should get their affairs in order because they had no more than a few months to live. But they found their way to a whole plant food lifestyle, and they lived and thrived for many years. One woman who had ovarian cancer says in the film her terminal cancer diagnosis, in which she was told she had only a few months left, "was eighteen years ago."

Eating You Alive shows what happens in a moving, dramatic way when people reverse chronic diseases for which they are told there is no cure, only remission. When people watch this captivating documentary, they laugh and cry, and their spirits rise with hope that there *is* a cure for disease that does not involve suffering. The projectionist in a movie theater where the film was shown wrote that she was so moved by the film that she promptly converted to a plant-based diet and lost 100 pounds in 8 months. Watch Eating You Alive and change your life.

EATING YOU ALIVE is a full-length documentary film owned by the Purjes Foundation, a charitable trust founded and privately funded by Dan and Edna Purjes. The film was made by SmallBox Entertainment. The filmmakers were Paul David Kennamer, director and producer, and Merrilee Jacobs, producer. Dan Purjes was the Executive Producer. **EATING YOU ALIVE can be rented or purchased at www.EatingYouAlive.com as well as on Amazon and iTunes.**

ACKNOWLEDGEMENTS

*We want to acknowledge and thank several people
who made this book possible.*

First and foremost, we want to express our deep gratitude to each storyteller for courageously sharing their inspiring story. This book would not have been possible without their contribution. We also want to thank our passionate editor, Colleen Greco Trovato, and our invaluable assistants, Mary Vitullo and Ross Licero, Jr. who worked tirelessly on the book. Also, Ian Serff of Serff Creative Gorup, our skilled designer and typesetter, Jennifer Tate of Earth & Sky Studios for graphic design, and Amit Peshwe and his digital marketing team at Exact Funnel. Abundant thanks to Paul David Kennamer , director and producer, and to Merrilee Jacobs, producer, of *DISEASE REVERSAL HOPE: The Film.*

Importantly, would like to thank the incomparable Dr. Caldwell Esselstyn, Jr. and his delightful wife, Ann, for their tenacious and contagious compassion to help people. And for introducing Dan and Scott to one another!

Finally, we wish to thank the pioneers of lifestyle medicine who envisioned a better way through a whole plant food lifestyle. They fought to lay a new foundation for medicine on which we stand today.

Dan Purjes & Scott Stoll, M.D.

ABOUT DAN PURJES

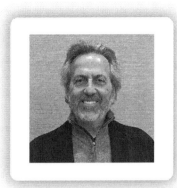

Dan Purjes is a successful entrepreneur and businessman, having built several companies to significant levels before selling them. These enterprises were in a variety of industries such as finance, technology, software, home automation, and solar energy. The funds from those activities have enabled him and his wife Edna ("Ed") to actively promote the message of health and disease reversal through a whole foods, plant-based diet. For more information, please visit **www.PurjesFoundation.org**.

Dan co-founded with Dr. Scott Stoll the *International Journal of Disease Reversal & Prevention*, a peer-reviewed scientific journal that publishes original research and other science-based articles on plant-based diets and disease reversal. He and Scott Stoll also co-founded the *Disease Reversal & Prevention Digest*, a periodical that presents in layman's language the science contained in the Journal.

Dan is the Executive Producer of the gripping documentary film, *Eating You Alive*, which is owned by the Purjes Foundation. He is also the Executive Producer of the documentary, Disease Reversal Hope: The Film, also owned by the Purjes Foundation, which will be released in early 2022.

Dan and his wife, Ed, have funded several plant-based scientific studies at major university hospitals. The funds for these studies came from their charitable trust, the Purjes Foundation, which is solely funded by Dan and Ed. Dan is on the Board of several non-profit organizations focused on plant-based health, including the Plantrician Project and the Ethos Farm Project. Dan arranged the merger of PlantBasedDocs.com, a division of the Plantrician Project, and PlantBasedDoctors.com; both competing companies provided directories of plant-based physicians and healthcare professionals. Their merger provided a more efficient directory.

Dan Purjes obtained a B.S. degree in Computer Science from the City College of New York, and an M.S. degree in Computer Science from the City University of New York. He completed all coursework for a Ph.D. in Computer Science at the University of Massachusetts, but did not complete a Ph.D. thesis. He went into business instead.

SCOTT STOLL, M.D., FABPMR

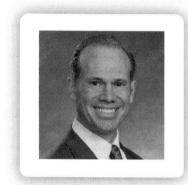

Dr. Scott Stoll graduated from the University of Colorado Medical School and completed his residency at the University of Colorado Hospital. For 16 years, he was an award winning physician in sports medicine and interventional spine health. Today, he is recognized as an international leader in lifestyle medicine and whole food, plant-based nutrition.

Scott is the Chairman and co-founder of the *Plantrician Project,* a non-profit organization with 20,000 physicians and healthcare professionals interested in the benefits of plant-based nutrition. He also established the *International Plant Based Nutrition Healthcare Conference,* the world's largest scientific healthcare conference devoted to plant-based nutrition. Scott co-founded the *International Journal of Disease Reversal & Prevention,* and the *Disease Reversal & Prevention Digest.* Scott also helped launch the Regenerative Health Institute, a unique collaborative project with the Rodale Institute that integrates a regenerative vision of human health, agriculture, and the environment.

Scott Stoll was a member of the 1994 Olympic Bobsled team. He served as a team physician for Lehigh University and also for the United States Bobsled and Skeleton Team. Scott served on the Google Food Lab board, and was a member of the Whole Foods scientific and medical advisory board.

In addition to authoring several books and numerous scientific articles, Dr. Stoll has appeared on a wide variety of national shows such as the Dr. Oz show. He hosted a 2018 PBS special, *Food As Medicine,* and was regularly featured in numerous documentaries including *Eating You Alive, Wait till it's Free, The Game Changers* and *Disease Reversal Hope: The Film.*

Every year Dr. Stoll hosts a very popular one-week total health immersion in Florida, helping attendees recover lost health, overcome addictions, and restore emotional balance. A passionate educator and sought-after international speaker, Dr. Stoll can be found on podcasts, and at conferences around the world, educating physicians and medical students about the power of lifestyle medicine. He is passionate about the ability of plant-based nutrition to prevent, suspend, and reverse disease.

And to restore hope.

COMING IN THE SPRING OF 2022

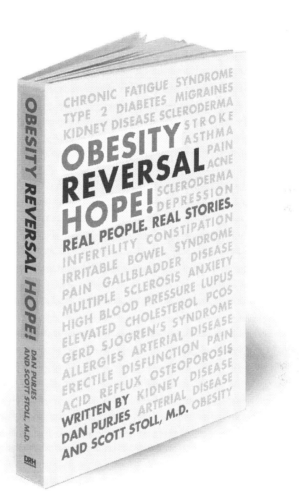

OBESITY REVERSAL HOPE!
Real People. Real Stories.

by Dan Purjes and Scott Stoll, M.D.

Send your email address and a note to
info@PurjesFoundation.org
to be notified when the book becomes available.

Made in the USA
Las Vegas, NV
31 January 2022

42719937R00151